The elderly

HANDBOOK ON CARE AND SERVICES

Published for the
NATIONAL OLD PEOPLE'S WELFARE COUNCIL
by
THE NATIONAL COUNCIL OF SOCIAL SERVICE
26 Bedford Square, London WC 1

Reference number 745
SBN 7199 0745 4

Age is Opportunity

Published	March 1949
Reprinted	May 1950
Revised	October 1952
New edition	March 1961

The elderly: handbook on care and services

New edition	March 1968

Printed by Blackfriars Press Limited, Leicester

Contents

Foreword

This is a handbook of up-to-date information on ageing and ways of caring for the elderly. It replaces *Age is Opportunity*, the previous handbook issued by the National Old People's Welfare Council. It is prepared for professional social workers, administrators, voluntary personnel and the medical profession, as well as for students. General readers will find much of interest too – for ageing is a process in which all share, and with which sooner or later everyone will be concerned.

It has been written by Mrs Pat Barr, and edited by Mr John Moss and Miss M. G. Wallis, to whom grateful thanks are recorded; as also to the Ministries of Health, Housing and Local Government, Social Security and others who kindly checked appropriate sections. The Council also gratefully acknowledges permission from the Controller of Her Majesty's Stationery Office to quote from Government publications.

Further reading is suggested at the end of each chapter. The *Quarterly Bulletin* issued by the National Old People's Welfare Council publishes regularly information about new developments research and latest publications.

December 1967

Special note

As this book goes to press the Health Services and Public Health Bill is before Parliament. If it becomes law it may affect the provision of certain services for the elderly which are mentioned in Chapters One, Three, Four, Five and Eight. Extracts from the Bill as published on 22nd November 1967 which are applicable to the care of the elderly, are given in the appendix.

Proposals were laid before Parliament on 16th January 1968 to introduce a charge of 2s 6d for prescriptions obtained under the National Health Service – men and women over 65, children under 15 and the chronic sick to be exempted; and also to raise the usual charge for dental treatment from £1 to £1 10s – those under 21, and nursing and expectant mothers to be exempted. People receiving supplementary benefits will have their charges met for them. Such arrangements will affect certain parts of chapters Two and Three.

February 1968

The elderly in our society

INTRODUCTORY

'I suppose one of the main difficulties of planning for the care of the aged is just this: "to respect their personalities while grouping their infirmities".' Eighty-year old Margery Fry said this at the International Gerontology Congress in 1954; the philosophy she defines is still with us. On the one hand there is a continuing increase in the number of elderly people in our society; in 1966 12·3% of our total population in England and Wales was above the age of 65 and by 1976 the percentage will have risen to 13·5. This does not mean that all these people will need help. Nevertheless, some will; and a larger number than at present will have reached the older age groups at which increasing infirmity and frailty, both physical and mental, occurs. In order to deal with these growing numbers, those responsible for the administration and operation of our social services must, to some extent, 'group the infirmities' of the aged, but old people are not simply the sum of their infirmities. Miss Fry put the case for us, 'to an administrator an individual may be just that old woman, I think her name is Jones, but to herself she is *the* Katie Jones who won a prize for Scripture and had the smallest waist in her class – with a thousand other distinctive features – who just happens to be old'. Everyone concerned in the well-being of the elderly in any way – those who plan national policies, those who administer them locally, those who provide personal care and practical aid on either a statutory or voluntary basis cannot afford to overlook this vital premise; we are all trying to help 'Mr and Mrs Katie Jones' who 'just happen to be old'.

But there is also this to remember. Age brings changes for the individual, and many of them are not pleasant. An old person's status and position in society alters radically on retirement; the physical structure and functions of the body are impaired with increasing age; powers of mental agility, sensory perception and emotional response all tend to decrease; sometimes degenerative diseases lead to increasing vulnerability and immobility. Old people need to make considerable physical, psychological and social adjustments in order to cope with these developments in their life cycle. Often it is not easy and old people are sometimes 'difficult' as a result. They need our understanding and comfort; we need their tolerance and patience.

Those working directly for old people try to minimise the adverse effects of these changes in all sorts of ways. They try to provide sheltered accommodation in which old people can live independently but with the knowledge that assistance is at hand if required; they bring various domiciliary services into the home so that old people do not have to expend all their failing physical energy on getting meals or cleaning the house; they provide companionship and leisure activities so that old people do not feel so isolated and cut off from the community. In all these and many other ways the service of volunteers is essential, for they can so often give the personal attention, the extra comfort and guidance which is so much needed. It has often been said that in the last analysis a society can be judged by the way it cares for its elderly and infirm members. If our society is to pass that test we must learn to use effectively, and in co-operation with each other, all our statutory and voluntary resources, to help those elderly who need it.

DEVELOPMENTS IN THE CARE OF THE ELDERLY IN OUR SOCIETY

BEFORE 1908

The history of welfare work for the elderly in Britain begins with voluntary effort. During the Middle Ages religious institutions of all kinds provided care for the old and infirm, the sick and needy, by providing food, clothing, money and shelter in almshouses, hostelries, or infirmaries. The Poor Law Act of 1601 placed the responsibility on each parish to care for its needy, many of whom were old. Overseers of the poor were appointed, a compulsory Poor Rate was instituted, and many parishes built dwellings to house the homeless. The first workhouses in which inmates contributed towards their keep by working were built in Bristol in 1697. During the next hundred years or so it became increasingly common for a parish to build its local workhouses to house its aged, mentally and physically handicapped, the unemployed and destitute. In 1834 a Poor Law Amendment Act was passed under which the parishes – some 15,000 – were grouped in 643 unions. The unions were controlled by elected Boards of Guardians whose officials – the Relieving Officers – enquired into and reported upon the conditions of the poor in their area. Outdoor relief (that is, that given outside the workhouse) was given to the sick and aged, widows and children; the 'able bodied' could only get relief by admission to a workhouse. This led to an increase in the number of these institutions, and conditions in them were generally deplorable.

Throughout this period voluntary effort to help the aged had continued. Parochial charities were established by local people and many country landowners provided aid or shelter for their aged tenants. Mutual aid through Friendly Societies began in the sixteenth century and became widespread and reasonably effective by the end of the period. A number of benevolent funds and trusts were founded which provided almshouse type accommodation or grants to people in particular groups (*see* chapter Two). New national undenominational organisations, in particular the British Red Cross Society and the St John Ambulance Brigade, were also founded at this time, and their members devoted a considerable amount of their effort towards helping the aged.

FROM 1908 TO 1940

The first Old Age Pensions Act was passed in 1908. It granted a non-contributory pension of five shillings per week to people over 70, subject to a means test and other conditions. In 1919 the maximum pension rate was raised to ten shillings; in 1925 the principle of social insurance was introduced in the form of contributory pensions. In addition to the new pension (which was given regardless of means), pensioners could apply for additional financial help under the Poor Law. The Boards of Guardians were abolished in 1930 and replaced by county and county borough councils acting through public assistance committees. The Ministry of Health, which had been established ten years earlier, was responsible for the oversight of this new scheme. During this period the accommodation provided for the elderly by local authorities was nearly always in the cheerless wards of workhouse buildings. Voluntary bodies were the first to recognise the urgent need for good, comfortable accommodation in smaller communal homes, and the earliest of these homes was opened by the Salvation Army in 1910. Other pioneers in this field were the Church Army, the Catholic and Anglican Sisterhoods, and the Free Churches.

FROM 1940 TO 1967

Statutory Development: In 1946 the Assistance Board became responsible for granting assistance through supplementary pensions (instead of through poor relief) to old age pensioners according to need. As a result three quarters of a million elderly applied for and received assistance who had not previously applied for poor relief, and the extent of real economic distress among the elderly in this country was clearly demonstrated. After the second world war three acts were passed which greatly affected the welfare of old people: the National Insurance Act (1946) set up the Ministry of Pensions and National Insurance and replaced the contributory old age pensions by retirement pensions to be paid on retirement from regular work; the National Health Services Act (1946) established comprehensive health and welfare services; the National Assistance Act (1948) established a comprehensive system of assistance for those in economic need, including responsibility for non-contributory pensions. Under the latter act county and county borough councils were made responsible for the provision of residential accommodation for 'persons who by reason of age, infirmity, or for any other circumstances are in need of care and attention which is not otherwise available to them'. Following this legislation a great many local authority homes for the elderly have been opened in all parts of the country to replace former public assistance institutions or workhouses although some of them still remain.

These acts provided the broad outline for the functioning of the 'Welfare State' throughout the 1950's; amendments and additions made to the working of the acts were generally in the direction of greater flexibility and extension of benefit and generosity to those in real need. In 1957 *A Survey of Services Available to the Chronic Sick and Elderly* (the Boucher report) was published by the Ministry of Health. This was followed by circular 14/57 which gave hospitals and welfare authorities the first central direction, placing responsibility for those infirm elderly not requiring hospital care on local authorities. A memorandum *Care of the Elderly in Hospitals and Residential Homes* issued in 1965 gave further direction to hospitals and local authorities on the division of their authority. In 1959 the National Insurance Act provided for a measure of additional graduated retirement pensions. During the 1950's the Ministry of Housing and Local Government re-examined the matter of housing the elderly. Housing authorities were asked to give particular thought to the needs of the elderly in their areas, to consider provision of certain special facilities and were reminded of the need to co-operate with voluntary organisations in this field. Section 56 of the Local Government Act (1958) empowered the county councils to make what payments they thought fit towards costs incurred by county district councils in the provision of special housing services for the elderly.

Overall trends in the operation of the statutory social services that emerged during the 1950's have been further developed by successive governments during the 1960's. Following the publication of the Ministry of Health's ten year hospital plan in 1962, local health and hospital authorities were asked to institute a ten-year development plan in their areas in close consultation with voluntary organisations; standard rates of pension were raised in 1963 and again in 1965 and 1967 (though this hardly keeps abreast of the rising cost-of-living index); the number of special housing units for the elderly provided by local authorities has continued to increase (though this still falls far short of overall needs). In 1966 the functions of the Ministry of Pensions and National Insurance and the National Assistance Board were combined and replaced by the Ministry of Social Security. Within the Ministry of Social Security there is a Supplementary Benefits Commission which is responsible for the administration of non-contributory benefits. It is the Ministry's present policy to eliminate the previous distinctions made between contributory and non-contributory benefits.

In 1966 the Committee on Local Authority and Allied Personal Social Services (Seebohm Committee) was set up. The Committee's published report is expected in 1968 and it may well recommend a new structure of social services as they affect the family.

Voluntary Development: During the last twenty-five years an increasing number of voluntary organisations have concentrated either all or part of their effort in helping the elderly. They range from large national societies with branches in various parts of the country to small independent local groups. Some of these are listed below. (For a description of the actual functions and organisation of the National Old People's Welfare Council in relation to old people's welfare committees, and the kind of help provided by them and individual voluntary organisations, *see* chapter Four.)

(1) *The National Old People's Welfare Council:* In 1940 a National Old People's Welfare Committee was established on the initiative of the National Council of Social Service. The committee was made up of some twenty national voluntary organisations, observers from government departments and individuals with special experience. The terms of reference of the National Old People's Welfare Committee were 'to study the needs of old people and to encourage and promote measures for their well-being'. The late Miss Eleanor Rathbone, MP, was the committee's first chairman; Sir Frederick Messer, CBE, MP, was chairman from 1946 to 1951; he was succeeded by Mr John Moss, CBE, who retired in 1967 when Mrs Denise Newman was appointed to succeed him. In 1955 the Committee changed its title to the National Old People's Welfare Council, as better suited to a co-ordinating body. The Council has its own constitution; the National Council of Social

Service acts as its trustees. Financially the Council depends on support from national appeals and donations from public bodies and private individuals; from grants from various Trusts, particularly the National Corporation for the Care of Old People and the Sembal Trust; and an annual grant from the Ministry of Health. The Council pays the National Council of Social Service for shared administrative services and the National Council of Social Service makes up any National Old People's Welfare Council deficit.

Since its inception up to the present day the Council has been a national focal point for information and advice, on all aspects of the care of the elderly. Like the local committees or associations for whom it acts as headquarters, the Council is independent, non-political and inter-denominational. It brings together in consultation at national level the principal bodies, both statutory and voluntary, concerned with the health and welfare of old people. It also maintains contact with foreign countries who have already established, or are in process of setting up voluntary organisations for the care of the elderly. Organisations not eligible for full membership of the Council and interested individuals may join its associate membership scheme, which entitles its members to appoint representatives to the Council. Soon after 1940 the Northern Ireland Council of Social Service, the Scottish Council of Social Service, and the Council of Social Service for Wales and Monmouthshire also formed old people's welfare committees which in their turn were quick to create public interest, and initiate and develop comprehensive services for the elderly in their countries. They act, as does the National Old People's Welfare Council, in combination with statutory and voluntary organisations, and their membership is widely representative of all those concerned in the field of welfare for the elderly. They co-operate and share information and experience with the National Old People's Welfare Council, on which they have representation.

Much of the specialised work and policy planning of the Council is carried out by its committees. Through these committees and the work of its full-time staff, the Council helps to create at national level, informed public opinion and hopes to actively encourage all efforts, whether statutory or voluntary, that are made to promote old people's well-being. The council also has an information service which records information of all aspects of old people's welfare; this is much used by official bodies and private individuals, both in this country and abroad.

Every two years the Council holds a National Conference on the care of the elderly which brings together delegates from all types of organisations, both statutory and voluntary, that are concerned in the work. By making approaches to, and consulting with, various government departments, the Council is able to play its part in national and local planning programmes that concern old people's welfare. The overall aim of the Council's varied activities is to provide for those elderly who need help a co-ordinated nation-wide service which makes effective use of both statutory and voluntary agencies.

(2) *National Corporation for the Care of Old People:* The National Corporation for the Care of Old People was founded in 1947 as an independent organisation by the Nuffield Foundation. Substantial funds were made available for the Corporation from the Nuffield Foundation and the Lord Mayor of London's National Air-Raid Distress Fund to allow for direct grants to voluntary organisations in all parts of the country which were providing accommodation and services for the elderly. In its early days the Corporation's main work was concerned with grant aid, but in recent years it has turned increasingly to study the changing needs and conditions of the elderly, and to undertake or stimulate research and experiment of all kinds in the field. The Corporation also collects information on what has been done or is being done for the elderly by statutory and voluntary bodies; it publishes an annual report, and from time to time publishes additional reports on particular aspects of old people's welfare. The Corporation works in close co-operation with the National Old People's Welfare Council on matters in which the two bodies share a mutual interest.

(3) *National Federation of Old Age Pensions Associations:* The National Federation of Old Age Pensions Associations was formed in Preston in 1940. It now has more than 1500 local branches and ninety area councils which are a very important part of the move-

ment. Although originally established to press for a higher retirement pension (and still actively concerned in obtaining better financial provision for retired people), the local associations have become increasingly interested in the general welfare of their members. Many run clubs and organise other social activities and are linked with old people's welfare committees. The Federation's headquarters have been established at Blackburn since 1947. It publishes a weekly journal *Pensioners' Voice*.

There is a separate organisation for Wales which is known as the National Old Age Pensioners Association of Wales.

(4) *British Geriatrics Society:* The word 'geriatrics', meaning the study of the treatment of diseases of the elderly, was first used by the American physician Nascher who published a treatise on diseases of old age in 1914. Gerontology means the study of ageing in its wider biological, psychological and social aspects. In Great Britain the increased interest of the medical profession in these fields was reflected in the formation of the Medical Society for the Care of the Elderly in 1947. Membership includes hospital physicians practising geriatrics, general practitioners, medical officers of health, medical administrators and research workers in university departments. In September 1959 the title of the society was changed to British Geriatrics Society, with the former name retained as a sub-title. There are now 460 members and the Society has formed nine regional groups in England, Scotland and Wales. Proceedings are published in *Gerontologia Clinica* which is the official journal of the Society.

(5) *Other national voluntary organisations concerned with the welfare of old people:* There are many national voluntary organisations concerned with the welfare of all age groups who have during the post-war years developed their services for the elderly as the needs of this group have become of paramount importance. Some of these organisations are represented on the National Old People's Welfare Council and on county and local committees, for example, the Women's Royal Voluntary Service, the British Red Cross Society, the St John Ambulance Brigade, Rotary International, Toc H etc. Others, such as the Royal National Institute for the Blind and the Royal National Institute

for the Deaf, and organisations dealing with particular illnesses are not as a rule specifically represented but there is usually a local link between officers so that individual elderly people can be helped when the need arises. (*See* chapter Four for further details about voluntary bodies.)

PREPARATION FOR RETIREMENT

In 1955 the National Old People's Welfare Council appointed a special study group to consider the whole question of Preparation for Retirement and to advise it as to any action which might be taken. A report of the findings of the group was published in 1959. In 1960 the National Corporation for the Care of Old People made a grant to the Council which enabled a full-time secretary to be appointed to its Preparation for Retirement Committee. In 1964 it was decided that 'Preparation for Retirement' would be better served by not being linked with old people's welfare and therefore in 1964 the Preparation for Retirement Committee became the Pre-Retirement Association, an independent organisation with its own constitution and legal entity as a charity. Until July 1966 the Association used 26 Bedford Square as its office but now has its headquarters at the National Institute of Adult Education. The Association has issued a number of useful publications. (For information about Pre-Retirement courses *see* chapter Eight.)

INTERNATIONAL DEVELOPMENTS

In countries abroad, concern about the welfare of the elderly has usually arisen in connection with medical needs. Pensions and social security schemes affecting the elderly are discussed internationally through the International Social Security Association, whose office is in Geneva. Some idea of the population of elderly people in various parts of the world is shown by the fact that, according to United Nations statistics for 1965, France, West Germany, Norway, Sweden, Belgium and the United Kingdom had more than eleven per cent of their total population aged sixty-five and over. This is an increase of approximately one per cent over the 1956 figures. Australia and the United States of America had over eight and nine per cent respectively in 1965.

The United Nations has understandably shown interest in the care of the elderly. In 1949 the Economic and Social Council of the United Nations, arising out of discussion at the Sixth Session of the Commission on Human Rights, had a report prepared by the Secretary General which appeared in January 1950. This summarised measures for the care of the elderly in a number of countries, including the United Kingdom, and was the first attempt at international documentation, even though it was on a limited scale from the point of view of scope and the number of countries concerned.

In 1955 the European office of the United Nations Technical Assistance Administration arranged the first of a series of seminars for representatives from European countries to discuss together the needs of the elderly. Seminars have now been held in Belgium, Germany, the United Kingdom and Sweden. The United Nations has also convened a number of seminars and study groups on other subjects closely connected with the welfare of the elderly which are of interest to those working in this field. More recently the International Labour Organisation has issued reports affecting the elderly and the World Health Organisation has sponsored fellowships so that some of those concerned with the care of old people can study the methods and services employed in other countries.

The International Association of Gerontology was formed in 1950. It convenes a congress every three years and the last one took place in Vienna in 1966. The accepted pattern now is to include both medical and social interests in the conference. Regional groupings, such as the European Social Research Section was set up in 1954. Others concerned with medical aspects help continuity between congresses and in some countries there are Gerontological Societies. The fact that Dr J. H. Sheldon, CBE, was President of the International Association for the period including the London congress has contributed towards the growth of interest in the social medicine of old age. Dr Sheldon's original work of 1947, *The Social Medicine of Old Age,* is well known internationally.

Dr A. L. Vischer, author of *On Growing Old,* was one of the earliest people to realise the importance of special medical care for the elderly. Switzerland's part in the early development of geriatrics may not always be recognised. Sweden has been the pioneer country in providing residential homes for the elderly and is now turning its attention to consideration of development of more domiciliary care. Sweden in fact also pioneered special training for wardens and matrons of homes for the elderly and their experience was extremely useful when such training was started in the United Kingdom in 1950. At the present time these two countries and several others in Europe have schemes of training for staffs of homes.

During recent years, there has been a continuing demand from overseas for information about developments in social work, particularly about domiciliary services and the idea of comprehensive care for the elderly in the United Kingdom. It is likely, therefore, that the experience of the United Kingdom has been useful in stimulating interest and activity abroad. A number of countries now have a national organisation similar in function to the National Old People's Welfare Council, for example Australia, the Netherlands, Norway and South Africa. Miss M. Bucke, the secretary of the United Kingdom National Old People's Welfare Council, at the invitation of the Australian National Old People's Welfare Council, has twice spent some weeks in that country in an advisory capacity. In Australia, New Zealand and South Africa work is being done through local co-ordinating old people's welfare committees formed on United Kingdom lines.

There is much interchange of knowledge between different parts of the world on all aspects of the care of the elderly. Many workers come to study United Kingdom methods and very many find their way to the office of the National Old People's Welfare Council to hear about the work and attitudes here and to see voluntary and other services in action. In 1966 and 1967 the Council organised two study tours abroad. The first was for matrons and assistant matrons of old people's homes who visited homes in Sweden and Norway. The second for secretaries and officers of old people's welfare committees who visited the Netherlands and saw a number of services for old people.

It is perhaps not untrue to say that the United Kingdom has been the pioneer in the idea of partnership between statutory and voluntary and medical and social interests – in fact, a partnership between all interests on a national and local level.

Nevertheless, it should not be assumed that the United Kingdom has nothing to learn from other countries. The opportunity for personal exchange of visits, and for international exchange afforded through the triennial congresses organised by the International Association of Gerontology, helps to stimulate and create new interest and new thinking for the benefit of the elderly throughout the world, as it is now evident that problems of old age are of world-wide concern, and achievements of the elderly of world-wide interest.

In judging, however, the achievements of any country in caring for its old people, it is important to know about the full range of services available in various parts of that country which may not necessarily be seen in the capital or the main cities. International understanding of the needs of the elderly depends on reliable knowledge of the background conditions, activities and policies of individual countries. This needs to be related to factual evidence of all the services and facilities provided for the elderly section of the community on a national and not only a local basis.

FUTURE TRENDS IN THE CARE OF THE ELDERLY

All welfare services for the elderly are at present short of two most precious commodities: money and staff. Unfortunately neither of these acute shortages is likely to be substantially alleviated during the next ten or even twenty years. It has been shown that in some areas present need can only be satisfactorily met by a doubling of present expenditure in the provision of domiciliary care, for example. Inevitably, and rightly too, as the benefits of services for the elderly, such as chiropody and meals services become more widely known, the demand for them will continue to expand, as the increasing numbers of the frail and infirm appreciate new possibilities of help.

In planning services now there is need to think of the increased numbers who will probably be using them in the future. Too often estimates of future expenditure allow for little more than the maintenance of the status quo. It is very important, therefore, that all those concerned with old people's welfare should be aware of present shortcomings as well as estimated future needs, so that planning can be adequate to cover both contingencies.

If the trend in the future is for local authorities to assume more overall responsibility for the welfare of our elderly citizens, this will not lessen the importance of the contribution of voluntary organisations. Each will have its own role to play and each will increasingly need the help and support of the other. It is of paramount importance today that statutory authorities and voluntary bodies should work together in a co-ordinated scheme and this may well become even more essential in the future when the numbers of very old people increase. On the other hand, the elderly of the future may be healthier and more affluent than the majority are today. If this is so the emphasis may then be on more housing schemes, day centres and domiciliary services than on residential accommodation.

If planning is to be adequate and realistic it needs to be far-sighted and to take into account that the elderly of the next century are likely to be very different from those of today. When buildings today have to be designed to last fifty or sixty years this is not easy, but it underlines the need for research and for co-ordinated planning by experts in many fields, medical, social, economic and architectural, to name but a few.

It has often been said that the degree of true civilisation a society has attained can be judged by the way it treats its old people; let us be sure that we are not condemned by later generations as barbarians.

REFERENCES

HMSO Publications:

Annual Reports of the Ministry of Housing and Local Government.

Annual Reports of the Ministry of Social Security.
Annual Reports of the Ministry of Health.
Health Services and Public Health Bill. 1967. 5s 9d

For further reading:

(*A*) NOPWC/NCSS *Publications:*
Old Age Looks at Itself, Margery Fry. Reprint of an address to the International Association of Gerontology, 1955, 1s 3d
Age Through the Ages. 1963, 1s 3d
Old People's Welfare Committees—Why They Are Needed: How They Are Started: What They Do. 1965, 1s 3d
Notes For Those Nearing and Over Sixty. 1966, 6d (Being revised)
Quarterly Bulletin of current information; issued March, June, September, December. 8d per issue (excluding postage) and annual subscription 4s 0d (including postage).
NOPWC *Biennial Conference Reports.* 5s 0d
NOPWC *Annual Reports.* 1s 6d
Visual Aid Material concerned with the Care of the Elderly. A list, 6d

(*B*) *Other Relevant Publications:*
The Aged in the Welfare State, P. Townsend and D. Wedderburn. 1965. G. Bell and Sons, 21s 0d
Living with Old Age, B. Ingleby and M. Yorath. 1966, Robert Hale, 15s 0d
Old and Alone, J. Tunstall. 1966, Routledge and Kegan Paul, 45s 0d
Social Administration and the Citizen, K. Slack. 1966, Joseph, 45s 0d
On Growing Old, A. Vischer. 1966, Allen and Unwin, 30s 0d
Ageing Process of Population, E. Rossett. 1964, Pergamon Press, 80s 0d
Understanding Old Age, R. Emery. 1967, National Association for Mental Health, 39 Queen Anne St, London W 1, 5s 0d
Social and Medical Problems of the Elderly, K. Hazell. 1965, Hutchinson, 50s 0d
The Process of Ageing, A. Comfort. 1965, Weidenfeld and Nicolson, 27s 6d
A New Look at Geriatrics, R. Kemp. 1965, Pitman, 7s 6d
The Practice of Geriatrics, J. Agate. 1963, Heinemann, 50s 0d
Annual Reports of the National Corporation for the Care of Old People, Nuffield Lodge, Regents Park, London NW 1
The Psychology of Human Ageing, D. Bromley. 1966, Pelican Books, 6s 0d
Social Policies for Old Age, B. Shenfield. 1957, Routledge and Kegan Paul, 25s 0d
Sans Everything, edited by B. Robb. 1967, Nelson, 18s 0d

The Family Life of Old People, P. Townsend. 1963, Penguin Books, 5s 0d
Facing Retirement, by a Country Doctor. 1964, Allen and Unwin, 18s 0d
The Clinical Psychiatry of Late Life, F. Post. 1965, Pergamon Press 21s 0d
Current Achievements in Geriatrics, W. F. Anderson and B. Isaacs. Conference report. 1964, Cassell, 30s 0d
Health and Happiness in Old Age, C. Westropp and M. Williams. 1960, Methuen, 8s 6d
Age and Function, A. Heron and S. Chown. 1967, J. & A. Churchill, 45s 0d
An Approach to Old Age and Its Problems, M. N. Hill. 1961, Oliver and Boyd, 15s 0d
The Ageing Countryman, H. C. Miller. 1963, National Corporation for the Care of Old People, 10s 6d
Old Age, A Register of Social Research, National Corporation for the Care of Old People. 1955-1964, 12s 6d; 1964 onwards, 20s 0d including future supplements.
The Last Refuge, P. Townsend. 1962, Routledge and Kegan Paul, 60s 0d. Abridged edition 1964, 30s 0d; Paperback abridged, 10s 6d
Parents Growing Old. The National Marriage Guidance Council, 58 Queen Anne St, London W 1, 1963, 2s 6d

Some Relevant Publications published abroad:

Group Work With Older People. 1963, National Association of Social Workers, New York. $2.75
Ageing in Western Societies, edited by E. W. Burgess. 1961, University of Chicago Press.
Growing Old—The Process of Disengagement. Cumming and Henry. 1961, Basic Books, New York, $6.75
Handbook of Social Gerontology, C. Tibbitts. 1960, University of Chicago Press, 90s 0d
A Classified Bibliography of Gerontology and Geriatrics, N. W. Shock. 1951, Stanford University Press, $15.00: Supplement I (1949-1955) $15.00: Supplement II (1956-1961) $10.00
Problems of Ageing, H. J. Loether. 1967, Prentice-Hall International, 16s 0d

Useful Addresses:

Addresses of all local old people's welfare committees can be obtained from: National Old People's Welfare Council,
26 Bedford Square, London WC 1

CHAPTER TWO

Financial position of the elderly

No person in the United Kingdom needs to be without a minimum source of income from the State or private source, or both. Possible sources of income are described below.

STATUTORY SOURCE

A retirement pension may consist of two parts: first, the flat rate pension which is paid in return for flat rate contributions (often called 'stamps'); second, graduated pension paid in return for contributions which are 'graduated', or graded, according to an employee's earnings over £9 a week.

FLAT RATE RETIREMENT PENSION

Most people below pension age are liable for *flat rate contributions* and can therefore expect to qualify for flat rate retirement pensions. A married woman is not obliged to pay flat rate contributions. If she does so she can qualify for a pension on her own insurance record; otherwise her entitlement to flat rate pension depends on her husband's record. The standard rate of pension for a married woman who relies on her husband's insurance is somewhat less than the rate for a person who has paid contributions. The standard rate of pension for a widow, however, is the same as for a contributor. Pension can be claimed, and notice of retirement given where necessary up to four months in advance by completing a form obtainable from the Ministry of Social Security. Payment of pension is usually made in advance by means of a weekly book of orders that can be cashed at a post office. Arrangements can be made for a pensioner to have his retirement pension paid quarterly in arrears by payable orders which can be paid into a bank account.

General conditions for receiving a flat rate retirement pension are:

(1) Minimum age is 65 for men and 60 years for women.

(2) Retirement from regular full time paid employment. The retirement condition ceases to apply at 70 for men and 65 for women. A person can be treated as having retired from full time employment even though he continues to work 'only occasionally' or 'to an inconsiderable extent' which is usually interpreted as meaning not more than twelve hours per week. He can also be treated as retired if his earnings are expected not to exceed, or only occasionally to exceed, the amount which would cause the pension, if awarded, to be reduced under the earnings rule (*see* 4 *below*).

(3) A total of 156 flat rate contributions must have been paid towards a pension. The contributions paid or credited (in weeks of sickness or unemployment) must average at least fifty a year for the standard rate of pension. If the yearly average is less than fifty, (but not less than thirteen) a reduced rate of pension is payable. Married women claiming on their own insurance must have paid or been credited with flat rate contributions for at least half the weeks between their date of marriage and sixtieth birthday. A married woman of sixty or over is treated as retired if she is engaged only in her home duties; but she does not receive a flat rate retirement pension on her husband's insurance unless he is entitled to his own pension.

(4) During the first five years after the minimum pensionable age the pension is subject to an earnings rule. This means that a person who has retired, but subsequently takes up work during this five year period, has his pension reduced or extinguished if his weekly earnings exceed an amount laid down in regulations. Retirement however need not be final and a pensioner under 70 (65 for a woman) who decides to resume work can cancel his pension and make contributions towards an additional pension later. A person can cancel his retirement on only one occasion.

Increases on basic flat rate pension:

(1) *For dependants* (*adults*): a pensioner can normally receive an increase of his pension for his wife, if she is living with him or he is maintaining her, whatever her age, provided she is not earning more than a fixed sum per week and is not herself entitled to receive a pension or any other benefit. Where a pensioner is not entitled to an increase for his wife he may be entitled to an increase for a woman who has the care of a child for whom he is entitled to benefit.

(2) A pensioner can claim a fixed allowance for *a child in his family,* or one whom he maintains; a lower allowance is payable for each subsequent child.

(3) *Working after retirement age:* A person who continues to work after the minimum pensionable age remains liable for national insurance contributions until the age of 70 (65 for a woman).

Pensioners who continue to work after the statutory retirement age and to pay full national insurance contributions, receive extra flat rate pensions when they ultimately retire. For every nine flat rate contributions actually paid for weeks of employment after pensionable age (from 30th October 1967), the pension is increased by one shilling, but weeks of sickness or unemployment do not count towards extra pension. A man between 65 and 70 (women 60 and 65) who has not retired, and who is entitled to receive a pension when he ultimately retires, can claim unemployment or sickness benefit in the ordinary way.

GRADUATED PENSION

This is paid in return for graduated contributions, for which employees over 18 and earning more than £9 a week are liable. Members of occupational pension schemes which satisfy certain requirements, however, can be contracted out of the graduated part of the national insurance scheme by their employers. The same conditions about age and retirement apply to graduated pension as to flat rate retirement pension; the amount payable depends on the total number of graduated contributions paid. Those who do not retire at minimum age may earn extra graduated pension as well as flat rate pension.

SUPPLEMENTARY PENSIONS

Those who are over pension age, and are not in full time work, have a statutory right to have their incomes brought up to a guaranteed weekly level. People who think they might qualify for this are encouraged to obtain a Claim Form (SP1) from the local office of the Ministry of Social Security or a post office. Claimants can be interviewed about their financial circumstances either at the Ministry's local office or in their own homes.

Qualifying conditions for supplementary pensions are:

(1) A person has reached statutory retirement age and is not in full time employment. For a married couple to qualify the husband must have reached the age of 65.

(2) In assessing weekly income, some sorts of income are taken into account in full; others are ignored, in full or in part. For example, retirement pension and most other national insurance benefits are counted in full, but at least the first £1 of the total of most other kinds of income is ignored, as well as the first £2 of any part time earnings. 'Income' also includes the 'tariff' income, which under statutory rules has to be taken into account in respect of capital.

The supplementary pension is the amount required to bring the assessed income up to the guaranteed weekly level. This consists of scale rates laid down by Parliament together with an allowance for rent or similar outgoings, and a standard addition to provide a margin for any special expenses. The supplementary pension may be increased if, exceptionally, the claimant has continuing special expenses, for example because of illness or disability, which amount to more than this standard addition.

(3) Those elderly people who formerly received non-contributory pensions now receive supplementary pensions automatically.

Additional Benefits

(1) Lump-sum payments to meet exceptional expenditure may be paid according to the particular circumstances of the claimant.

(2) Persons in receipt of supplementary pensions are entitled to receive help with the cost of national health services, charges for glasses, dentures and dental treatment.

WAR PENSIONS

A person receiving a war disablement pension is entitled to a retirement pension if he satisfies the normal qualifying conditions, but retirement pension cannot be paid in addition to a war pension unemployability supplement or severe disablement occupational allowance. The wife of a war pensioner can receive a retirement pension on his insurance provided that all the age, retirement and contribution conditions are satisfied, even if he is receiving an unemployability supplement or severe disablement occupational allowance. A retirement pension paid to the wife of a war pensioner on his insurance does not affect the wife's allowance paid with the basic war pension, but it extinguishes the additional wife's allowance paid with unemployability supplement. Those drawing a war pension, or war widow's pension, may also be entitled to supplementary pensions if their income falls below the weekly level guaranteed by the Ministry of Social Security, or even, in certain cases, if the weekly income is above this level. For further information about supplementary pensions or war pensions, enquire at one of the Ministry's local offices.

DEATH GRANTS

For those within ten years of pension age (65 for a man, 60 for a woman) when the national insurance scheme started on 5th July 1948, the grant is at half the standard rate. No death grant is payable for a man born before the 5th July 1883 or a woman born before the 5th July 1888. The Ministry of Social Security will provide information about whether or not there is an entitlement to a death grant (this depends on the age of the deceased and the number of national insurance contributions that had been paid).

SPECIAL CIRCUMSTANCES THAT AFFECT THE PAYMENT OF PENSIONS AND BENEFITS

Pensions in hospitals and institutions: Retirement pensions continue to be paid for the first eight weeks of a person's stay in hospital unless a patient has been transferred from another hospital or from a local authority home, or has returned to hospital again after a very short interval. After eight weeks a pensioner who is in hospital under the National Health Service has his pension paid at a reduced rate. The amount of reduction depends on whether or not the pensioner concerned has any dependants. When single claimants, or one of a married couple in receipt of a supplementary pension enters hospital, the pension is adjusted after a time if outside financial commitments are reduced, but all pensioners are entitled to be left with a certain fixed sum per week to meet personal needs. If pensioners who live in old people's homes run by local authorities, or by certain voluntary organisations, do not have sufficient income (as guaranteed by the Ministry of Social Security scales) to pay the minimum charge and be left with this fixed sum they are entitled to supplementary pension or allowance.

Pensioners abroad: National insurance retirement pensions can be paid anywhere in the world, subject only to certain currency restrictions for temporary absence outside the sterling area. The rate of pension payable is normally restricted to the rate payable when the pensioner leaves Great Britain to live abroad, or the rate for which he qualifies while living abroad. A pensioner who intends to be absent abroad for up to three months can ordinarily let his pension accrue and cash the orders on return to this country. Those who are uncertain about the duration of their absence abroad, or who intend to be away for longer than three months, should consult their local office of the Ministry of Social Security before their departure. Certain countries have reciprocal agreements on social security with the United Kingdom, some of which modify the general provision about the rate of pension payable abroad and may allow residence or contributions to the social security scheme in the other country to be taken into account. For further information, enquire at one of the Ministry's local offices.

PRIVATE PENSION SCHEMES

An increasing number of firms and industrial enterprises make individual arrangements for pension schemes for their employees. The size of contributions paid, both by employer and employee, and the resulting amount of pension payable on retirement, vary considerably. Such schemes do not usually cover employees in small firms or casual workers. Arrangements can sometimes be made to transfer superannuation rights by those changing their place of employment.

ASSURANCE

Assurance can be arranged during the years prior to retirement to provide a lump sum or a regular income on retirement, or a lump sum on death. Personal pensions are often arranged by those who, for various reasons – such as being self-employed – do not belong to occupational pension schemes. A number of accredited companies offer assurance policies and when taking out a policy factors such as the amounts of premium and bonuses and possibilities of income tax relief should be considered.

BENEVOLENT FUNDS OR CHARITABLE TRUSTS

A number of Funds and Trusts exist to help elderly people who meet their qualifying conditions. Aid can take the form of a small regular allowance, a lump sum payment for a particular purpose, and/or provision of accommodation. Details of charities, their purpose and administration, can be found in the Annual Charities Digest, Kelly's Directories, or the index maintained by the Charity Commissioners. Citizens' advice bureaux may also be able to give information on local charities.

Funds and Trusts fall broadly into the following categories:

GENERAL CHARITABLE ASSOCIATIONS

There are a few associations which operate on a national basis to give aid to elderly people, usually from a professional background, who are suffering particular hardship. Examples are: The Royal

United Kingdom Beneficent Association; The Elderly Invalids Fund; and the Distressed Gentlefolks' Aid Association.

TRADE OR PROFESSIONAL FUNDS

There are a number of these funds which give financial help or private residential accommodation to those applicants (or wives of applicants) who have been connected with a particular trade or profession. Examples of these are: military service regimental funds, funds for elderly nurses, and for retired teachers. Also Linen and Woollen Drapers Institution and Whiteley Homes Trust.

CHARITIES FOR PARTICULAR GROUPS

Some charities are administered by religious organisations to help primarily members of their particular denominations. For example, Methodist Homes for the Aged; there are also some associations which give help, either financially or with accommodation and other problems for sufferers from particular diseases or handicaps – for example, The British Rheumatism and Arthritis Association; Royal National Institute for the Blind; Royal National Institute for the Deaf.

LOCAL TRUSTS AND FUNDS

The benefits from some charities are restricted to those who live and/or have worked in a certain locality. Information about these can usually be obtained from the clerk of the county council or the town clerk.

INCOME TAX AND THE ELDERLY

Certain special tax reliefs are given to persons over 65. For full information about these, applications should be made to the tax inspector of the area.

In general, OCCUPATIONAL PENSIONS AND MINISTRY OF SOCIAL SECURITY PENSIONS are treated as income for tax purposes and are chargeable to tax under the normal rules if the total income from them and any other source is large enough to incur tax liability. It is important to inform the local tax office before retirement of impending receipt of a Ministry of Social Security pension. This prevents accumulation of tax arrears becoming payable after retirement. Pensions paid by employers may be taxed at source under PAYE. Those who retire and then resume work later on either on a full or part-time basis should inform their tax office as this may affect their tax position. If the pensioner's wife has a pension from a former employer or if she is entitled to a National Insurance pension *by virtue of her own contributions* the additional wife's earned income allowance may be due on it; such a pension will often be fully covered by the allowance. A pensioner may also be liable to pay tax on a proportion of the income from a purchased life annuity and the whole of any annuity from a former employer's pension scheme.

Tax is not payable on the value of a house in which the pensioner lives but if he lets part of it, he is liable to pay tax on rent received.

TAX RELIEFS FOR PERSONS OVER 65

Age exemption: If either a husband or wife is 65 or over, their total joint income is exempt from tax if it does not exceed £643 per year. Single people over 65 (living alone) are exempt if their income is not more than £401 a year. Persons whose income is slightly above these figures sometimes qualify for marginal tax relief. Age exemption applies only to those whose income is below these levels; not to all people over 65.

Age Relief: Those over 65 whose income is not more than £900 a year are entitled to a special allowance of two-ninths of any income from investments – for example, dividends on shares in a company. In general pensions count as earned income and already receive the two-ninths earned income allowance. Those whose income is a little more than £900 a year may qualify for marginal relief.

Relief for help in the home: A widow or widower who employs a housekeeper can claim an allowance for her.

An allowance can also be claimed if a daughter is living with and is maintained by an elderly parent and where her services are necessary on account of age or infirmity. A person who is old or infirm may be entitled to an allowance if he maintains a daughter who lives in his home to look after him. A married man is not entitled to this allowance unless his wife is old or infirm. This allowance is an alternative to the housekeeper allowance – it is not possible to claim both.

Other allowances: There is a special allowance for registered blind persons. There is also an allowance for those who maintain an aged or infirm relative, and this includes elderly parents who maintain an adult son or daughter who, because of physical or mental disability, cannot be employed. The amount of the allowance will depend on individual circumstances and information should be obtained from local tax offices.

Post-war credits: Men over 60 and women over 55 can claim repayment of any post-war credits to which they are entitled. Claim forms are available at any post office or income tax office.

OTHER FINANCIAL MATTERS

CONCESSIONS

Some local authorities allow retirement pensioners, along with certain other groups of the community, to travel at reduced rates on their public transport.

WILLS

It is in the interest of all adult persons, most particularly those over the age of 60, to make a will. Those who have even a small amount of capital or any other assets, such as property, are advised to see a lawyer about this in order that their wishes will be carried out and to eliminate possible complications for their survivors.

REMISSION OF RATES

See chapter Five.

REFERENCES

Circulars and other HMSO Publications:

Ministry of Social Security produces leaflets regularly on the following topics:

Retirement Pensions and other payment arrangements.
National Insurance.
Supplementary Pensions for those over retirement age.
Widows' Pensions and Benefits.
War Pensions and Treatment Allowances for the War Disabled.
Hospital Patients—reductions of certain benefits.
Death Grant and National Insurance Matters arising on a death.
Earnings Rule.

(All the most recent editions of these are available from the Ministry of Social Security local offices free).

Income Tax and the Elderly. Board of Inland Revenue. 1967. HMSO, *Free*

The Question of the Earnings Limit for Retirement Pensions. Report of the National Insurance Advisory Committee. 1967. HMSO, 3s 0d

Financial and other Circumstances of Retirement Pensioners. Ministry of Pensions and National Insurance. 1966. HMSO, 20s 0d

Everybody's Guide to Social Security. 1967. HMSO, 1s 0d

Annual Report of the Charity Commissioners. HMSO, 4s 6d

For further reading:

(*A*) NOPWC/NCSS *Publications:*

Notes for Those Nearing and Over Sixty. 1966, 6d (Being revised)

Annuities for the Retired:

Leaflet 1—Notes for the Retired Person. 3d
Leaflet 2—Explanatory Notes. 6d

(*B*) *Other relevant publications:*

The Economic Circumstances of Old People, D. Cole and J. Utting. 1962, Occasional Papers on Social Administration no 4, Codicote Press, 12s 6d

The £.s.d. of Retirement, C. Chisholm. 1957, Penguin, 3s 6d

Employment, Income and Retirement Problems of the Aged, edited by J. M. Kreps. 1964, Cambridge University Press, 60s 0d

Social Security and Pension Practice in Western Europe, Noble Lowndes Group. 1964, International Pension Consultants, 32 Lowndes St, London SW 1, *Free*

Social Security in Britain—A History, H. E. Raynes. 1957, Pitman, 30s 0d

The Aged in the Welfare State, P. Townsend and D. Wedderburn. 1965. Occasional Papers in Social Administration no 14, G. Bell and Sons, 21s 0d

Practical Problems Following the Death of a Relative or Friend. CAB leaflet. 1964, NCSS, 10 for 1s

Annual Charities Register and Digest. Family Welfare Association, 18s 6d

Living Arrangements and £.s.d., Lorna Hubbard, 1966, Pre-Retirement Association, 35 Queen Anne St, London W 1, 3s 6d

Directory of Grant-Making Trusts. Charities Aid Fund, NCSS, 1968, 85s 0d

Useful Addresses:

Board of Inland Revenue,
Somerset House, London WC 2

Ministry of Social Security,
6 St Andrew Street, London EC 4

Elderly Invalids Fund,
10 Fleet Street, London EC 2

Family Welfare Association,
296 Vauxhall Bridge Road, London SW 1

Charity Commission,
14 Ryder Street, London SW 1

National Citizens Advice Bureaux Council,
26 Bedford Square, London WC 1
(local CAB addresses can be obtained from this address)

CHAPTER THREE

Services provided by the National Health Service

INTRODUCTORY

The structure of the National Health Service falls into three parts each of which bears some responsibility for the care of the elderly:

(1) Services administered by local executive councils. These include general practitioner services, dental, supplementary ophthalmic and pharmaceutical services.
(2) Services administered by regional hospital boards, boards of governors of teaching hospitals and hospital management committees. These are hospital and specialist services.
(3) Services administered by local health authorities. These include many of particular concern to the elderly such as health visiting, home nursing, provision of ambulances and mental after care.

SERVICES ADMINISTERED BY LOCAL EXECUTIVE COUNCILS

GENERAL PRACTITIONER SERVICE

From the patient's point of view the family doctor is the key figure in the National Health Service. Nearly all other services are obtainable through him. It is, therefore, essential that every elderly person should be registered with a doctor. Application to be put on his list can be made directly to the doctor of one's choice; alternatively, lists of doctors providing general medical services in the National Health Service may be seen at any main post office. A person who moves to another address may take his medical card to a doctor in his new locality. Anyone who needs medical treatment while away from home can go to any local doctor in the service and be treated as a temporary resident without charge. A patient may change his doctor at any time by obtaining the consent of his present doctor – such consent being written, signed and dated on the patient's medical card. If he prefers, a patient may send his card to the local executive council with a letter stating his intention to transfer. He will be able to transfer fourteen days after the council receive his letter.

Treatment, medicines and dressings (including items such as elastic stockings and incontinence pads) are obtainable through the doctor and are prescribed free of charge. It is through a doctor that a patient can be admitted to hospital. A doctor can also arrange an appointment with a consultant or surgeon who may order the fitting of a surgical appliance such as a surgical boot or truss; these can be obtained free in certain instances. A doctor can also arrange for a nurse to call regularly to give domicilary treatment and care to a housebound patient, he can recommend certain cases to local authority officers or voluntary organisations for continuing or additional domiciliary services, for example home help, meals on wheels. Some doctors pay visits to all their patients over a certain age at regular intervals to make sure that their condition is not deteriorating.

OPHTHALMIC SERVICE

It is important for elderly people to have their eyes tested at least every two years. Those who have not previously had this done must obtain from their doctor a recommendation to see an ophthalmic medical practitioner or optician. Any subsequent testing or provision of spectacles may be obtained from the optician without a prior visit to the doctor. Moderate charges are made for spectacle lenses and frames are charged for according to the type supplied.

HEARING AIDS

Elderly people who become hard of hearing should be encouraged to see their doctor first to arrange for an appointment with a specialist. If a hearing aid is necessary the specialist will then recommend this. The Medresco Aids, which are of various types, are obtainable free under the National Health Service. If an aid develops a fault it should be returned at once to the Hearing Aid Clinic where it was obtained. (Addresses of these clinics are in the booklet issued with the aid.) The Royal National Institute for the Deaf offers free advice on the use of aids and a free testing service for aids which consistently cause difficulty.

DENTAL SERVICES

The dentist is the only practitioner in the National Health Service who may be consulted without introduction from a doctor. Persons wanting treatment under the National Health Service should make this clear at the time they seek an appointment with the dentist of their choice. Lists of dentists taking part in the service can be seen on request at main post offices and public libraries. Most routine treatments are available at a cost not exceeding one pound; additional charges are made for the fitting of dentures. In certain circumstances the Ministry of Social Security can help with the payment of these charges. In 1964 the Ministry of Health published a pamphlet entitled *Your Guide to Dental Treatment under the National Health Service*. This aims to make patients better aware of services available to them.

SERVICES ADMINISTERED BY REGIONAL HOSPITAL BOARDS, BOARDS OF GOVERNORS OF TEACHING HOSPITALS, AND HOSPITAL MANAGEMENT COMMITTEES

HOSPITAL AND SPECIALIST SERVICES

Introductory: In September 1965 the Ministry of Health issued a memorandum setting out the principles to which hospital boards and local authorities should refer when reviewing their development plans on the hospital geriatric services and care of the elderly, *Care of the Elderly in Hospitals and Residential Homes*. The memorandum defined more fully the respective responsibilities of hospital boards and local authorities and urged the need for continuing joint consultation and planning between the two services. In this the regional hospital boards were asked to take the initiative. In the actual operation of services, such as emergency allocation of beds and general assessment of need, the memorandum recommends close co-operation between all those concerned – the geriatrician, the geriatric social worker, the general practitioner and the health and welfare staff of the local authority.

With regard to the special responsibilities of hospital authorities in the care of the elderly, the memorandum stated that they should aim to provide as soon as practicable in every area an effective hospital geriatric service. To be effective, a hospital geriatric service should ensure that:

(1) Elderly people can be promptly admitted to hospital when the need arises.
(2) Their needs are fully assessed at the outset, preferably prior to admission.
(3) They are discharged in consultation with general practitioners and any local authority staff concerned so that preparations for after care are made and known.

Types of hospital care: An elderly patient can receive hospital care in any of the following ways according to his individual needs:

(1) *A general hospital:* An elderly patient who develops an acute illness can be admitted to the acute ward of the general hospital.

(2) *A geriatric unit:* Patients are admitted to such a unit for assessment followed by rehabilitation. Some patients requiring continuous nursing will be admitted for long-term care, as will others who have failed to respond to rehabilitation. Some patients will be admitted for terminal care.

Rehabilitation aims to restore the maximum degree of activity directed at re-establishing the patient's physical, mental, and social independence. This involves the work of a team; besides a doctor and nursing staff, the medical social worker, the physiotherapist, and occupational therapist and others play an important part in formulating and conducting an overall plan of treatment. Geriatric outpatient services attached to these units provide facilities both for consultation and for follow-up of patients discharged from hospital.

(3) *Long-stay hospital:* Those patients who are in need of continuing long-term care may be transferred to long-stay beds either within the general hospital or in a special annexe or peripheral hospital. It is desirable that long-stay accommodation is located and planned so that patients are able to maintain close links with family and friends wherever possible.

(4) *Day hospital:* An increasing number of elderly people now attend hospitals as 'day patients'. This means regular attendance at the hospital as part of a planned course of treatment; but day patients return home at night. Care of this sort may include such treatments or services as physiotherapy, the provision of special meals, chiropody, bathing and general medical supervision.

(5) *Temporary admission to hospital:* Elderly people in need of continuous care are sometimes admitted to geriatric hospitals for short periods to relieve their relatives. This is to assess their medical and social capabilities and to relieve their relatives in time of stress.

(6) *Psychiatric Hospitals:* Treatment for mental disorder is provided as part of the National Health Service. If mental disorder occurs in an elderly patient his doctor may, in consultation perhaps with a psychiatrist, a psychiatric social worker, or a consultant in geriatric medicine, arrange for hospital admission. If a patient is willing to undergo treatment, he may be admitted to a suitable hospital informally. In certain extreme circumstances if it is in the interests of the patient himself or society, mentally disordered people can be compulsorily detained in hospital; in general, compulsory powers are used very sparingly nowadays. Application for compulsory admission, which must normally be supported by the written recommendation of two medical practitioners, is regulated in England and Wales by the Mental Health Act, 1959. The application may be made by the patient's nearest relative or a mental welfare officer. Mental Health Review Tribunals exist to protect the patient from unwarranted detention.

SERVICES ADMINISTERED BY LOCAL HEALTH AUTHORITIES

INTRODUCTORY

The authorities responsible for health and welfare services are the councils of counties, county boroughs, London boroughs and the City of London. These authorities often work in co-operation with voluntary organisations to which they can make grants, lend premises, or give help in other ways. Their aim is to prevent illness and provide care and after-care to all those suffering from illness or mental disorder.

DOMICILIARY SERVICES provided by local authorities are available to elderly people as to members of the population generally. No service, either domiciliary or otherwise, is provided solely for the elderly, although their needs constitute the main demand of such services as home helps and home nurses. This demand is likely to continue as it is now generally recognised that the elderly should be encouraged to remain in their own homes as long as possible. Domiciliary health and welfare services are planned to help them in this. In practice, many of these services, for example night attendance and laundry services, are supplemented a great deal by voluntary effort.

The main services are as follows:

Home nurses: The home nurse is available without charge to visit the sick in their homes. Home nurses (or district nurses) are on the staff of the local health authority, but they carry out their duties at the request of a family doctor and are under his clinical direction. Home nurses give treatment, including injections and dressings, and can be of great help in giving advice to relatives on simple ways to augment the nursing care which they themselves provide. Many local authorities also employ nursing auxiliaries and lay assistants to help skilled nursing personnel. Useful articles for those nursing at home, such as bed pans, bed rests and feeding cups can be borrowed from the health department of a local authority, alternatively, application can be made to various voluntary organisations (*see* chapter Four).

Health visitors: The health visitor employed by the local health authority is concerned with the well-being of a family – even if the family consists of only one person. Her main function is the promotion of good health through health education and based on her knowledge of the home background. She makes it her business to visit and advise old people (among others) on matters concerning, for example, the prevention of accidents, general diet, and personal health matters; she may also arrange for other or additional domiciliary services to be provided. Voluntary organisations can apply to her direct or through the medical officer of health, for advice about health problems of those in their care. Her services are free.

Home Helps: In a circular sent in 1965 to county and county boroughs and the London boroughs concerning the working of the home help services it was suggested that authorities should undertake local studies in order to assess needs and review their services and plans realistically. Authorities were reminded of their right to impose charges for the services where reasonable, but were asked not to make a charge for provision of home helps to people in receipt of supplementary benefits or on an equivalent level of income. The home help service is intended to give a measure of essential domestic assistance (especially house work) to those who are incapacitated and cannot rely on the help of a relative. The amount of help needed is assessed by home help organisers who supervise the services in an area and recruit and deploy staff.

Night Attendance: Some local authorities provide for special home help or home nurses to be in attendance at night to look after old people who are very ill, or to relieve the strain on relatives. This is often carried out in conjunction with a voluntary organisation.

Laundry Services: Laundry services are organised by almost half the local authorities to help meet the extra needs of old people, in cases of long illness or infirmity where the patient is incontinent. Such services are run in conjuction with, or in addition to, services provided by voluntary organisations. Laundry facilities are usually restricted to the washing of soiled bed-linen, and authorisation from the medical officer of health or other professional worker is necessary before the service can be given.

Mental Care and After-Care: Local authorities have a duty to make arrangements for helping the mentally disordered in the community, and for their care and after-care. Mental welfare officers give advice and support to families looking after a mentally disordered person and to mentally confused old people living alone. Recent developments in the treatment of mental illness stress the desirability of discharging patients from a mental hospital in cases where it is felt that they can best benefit from living normal lives with the community.

This means that there is an increasing need for the services of mental health social workers, health visitors, psychogeriatric social workers, home helps and others who provide domiciliary help and support. In the case of the elderly it is particularly difficult to devise and enforce clear-cut criteria for mental health, as forgetfulness, lack of concentration, garrulity, and eccentricity are common in varying degrees among the over-seventies. The term 'mentally frail' is often used to describe this condition; but there could be a great divergence of opinion about the degree of confusion considered abnormal. In any case it is known that mental health among the elderly is to a greater extent than in any other group linked with physical and social health; therefore care and after-care services which help the old person to remain integrated members of the community are particularly valuable and necessary.

OTHER SERVICES PROVIDED BY LOCAL AUTHORITIES

The following are of particular concern to the elderly:

CHIROPODY

In 1959 the Ministry of Health authorised local health authorities to develop chiropody services, and suggested that priority be given to the elderly, the physically handicapped and expectant mothers.

Clinics could be held in suitable premises or in the chiropodist's own premises. Approval was given to the fixing of reasonable charges having regard to the means of the patient. In 1962 chiropodists obtained state registration under the terms of the Professions Supplementary to Medicine Act, 1960; and with certain exceptions only state registered chiropodists can be employed by local health authorities. On occasions local authorities contribute to the funds of voluntary organisations such as old people's welfare committees which are already providing chiropody services (*see* chapter Four). The district nurse, health visitor, general practitioner or voluntary visitor will give details of how and where chiropody services may be obtained locally.

AMBULANCE SERVICE

Free conveyance by ambulance is provided between home and hospital by local authorities either directly or by arrangement with voluntary organisations. Requests for the use of ambulance services must be made by a doctor or by a hospital except in the case of emergency or accident.

DAY CENTRES FOR THE ELDERLY AND THE YOUNGER HANDICAPPED

A Day Centre, as distinct from a club, caters primarily for the frail who are often partially house-bound or isolated. 120 of these had been established by the end of 1966 by local authorities. Special transport to them is usually necessary and a main mid-day meal is usually provided. The centres are staffed according to local needs, and a great deal of work is done by volunteers who help with administration, driving, preparing meals, and giving personal care and support.

ADVISORY HEALTH CLINICS

A small number of local authorities in co-operation with hospital authorities and general practitioners have provided advisory health clinics or centres for the elderly. Their object is to detect early onset of disease, maintain health and advise on particular social problems which some elderly people face.

WELFARE SERVICES FOR THE PHYSICALLY HANDICAPPED

The major local authorities have a duty to provide welfare services for those who are blind, partially sighted, hard of hearing, deaf, or otherwise substantially and permanently handicapped. The registers for all classes of handicapped people show a significant increase in the number of elderly people in this category. A wide range of facilities is provided by these services: help in carrying out adaptations in the home to alleviate the effects of the disability, social and occupational centres, advice on social and personal problems arising from the disability, and provision of special aids such as emergency call systems and white walking sticks.

REMOVAL OF PERSONS NEEDING CARE AND ATTENTION

A person who is 'suffering from grave chronic disease or, being aged, infirm or physically incapacitated' and is therefore unable to take proper care of himself and is not receiving it from others may, by Court order, be removed to a hospital or 'other suitable place'. Application for such an order may be made to a court of summary jurisdiction by the local authority on receiving a written report from the medical officer of health that such removal is in the person's interest or that his condition is causing injury to the health, or is a serious nuisance to other persons. Fortunately the need for exercising these compulsory powers does not arise frequently.

REFERENCES

Circulars and other HMSO Publications:

National Health Service Act, 1946. HMSO, 7s 6d

Mental Health Act, 1959. HMSO, 11s 0d

Chiropody Services. Ministry of Health Circular 11/59, *Free*

A Hospital Plan for England and Wales 1962. HMSO Cmnd. 1604, 18s 6d

Development of Local Authority Health and Welfare Services. Ministry of Health Circular 2/62, *Free*

Health and Welfare. The Development of Community Care. 1963, HMSO, Cmnd. 1973. 24s 0d (Revision to 1973-74, 22s 6d; Revision to 1975-76, 37s 6d).

Your Guide to Dental Treatment under the National Health Service. 1964. Ministry of Health leaflet, *Free*

The Local Authority Welfare Services. National Health Service note 7, 1964, *Free.*

Development of Local Authority Health and Welfare Services. Ministry of Health Circular 10/64, *Free*

Care of the Elderly in Hospitals and Residential Homes. Ministry of Health Memorandum 8/65, *Free*

Health Services and Public Health Bill, 1967. HMSO, 5s 9d

For further reading:

(*A*) NOPWC/NCSS *Publications:*

Notes for Those Nearing and Over Sixty. 1966, 6d (Being revised)

Statutory and Voluntary Services (Charts on a four-page card) 9d

(*B*) *Other relevant publications:*

Social Policies for Old Age, B. Shenfield. 1957, Routledge and Kegan Paul, 25s 0d

Social Administration and the Citizen, K. Slack. 1966, Michael Joseph, 45s 0d

Local Health and Welfare Services, J. Parker. 1965, Allen & Unwin, 25s 0d

The Day Hospital Movement in Great Britain, J. Farndale. 1961, Pergamon Press, 84s 0d

The Aged in the Welfare State, P. Townsend and D. Wedderburn. 1966, Occasional Papers on Social Administration no 14, G. Bell & Sons, 21s 0d

Guide to the Social Services, Family Welfare Association, Denison House, 296 Vauxhall Bridge Road, London SW 1; revised annually, 8s 6d

Consumer's Guide to the British Social Services, P. Willmott. 1967, Penguin Books, 6s 0d

Public Social Services, NCSS; revised 1965, 16s 0d

A New Look at Medicine and Politics, Enoch Powell. Pitman Medical Publishing Company, 7s 6d

Trends in Psychogeriatric Care. 1966, PEP, 7s 6d

A Guide to the State Eye Services. The Association of Optical Practitioners, 65 Brook Street, London W 1 (*Leaflet*)

Useful addresses:

Ministry of Health,
Alexander Fleming House, Elephant and Castle, London SE 1

Ministry of Social Security,
6 St Andrew Street, London EC 4

Royal National Institute for the Deaf,
105 Gower Street, London WC 1

Royal National Institute for the Blind,
224 Great Portland Street, London W 1

CHAPTER FOUR

Voluntary care of the elderly

INTRODUCTORY

VOLUNTARY PRINCIPLE IN THE CARE OF THE ELDERLY

Basic services for the elderly are provided by central and local government departments, but there is a constant and ever increasing need for a reservoir of voluntary help to supplement state provision. In this way it is possible to provide a comprehensive pattern of care in which voluntary workers enhance and augment the services of professional social workers. Well-organised voluntary services can utilise to the best effect the energies and enthusiasms of those members of the community – young, middle-aged, and elderly – who are willing to give part of their time to help others.

Moreover in the United Kingdom a traditional method of developing social services has been for the voluntary body to explore the possibilities of a service or pioneer it, and then for statutory authorities to take it over when its usefulness has been sufficiently proved for it to be supported from the public purse. This pioneering function of voluntary bodies has encouraged initiative and flexibility in the planning of social service policies.

VOLUNTARY WORKERS

In the past there were fewer voluntary helpers but individually they often had considerable time to devote to voluntary activities; nowadays many more offer to help, though they may only have two or three hours a week to spare. In these circumstances there is an even greater need for experienced and trained volunteers who are able to give considerable time to help in the administration and organisation of voluntary effort. Wherever possible it is desirable that volunteers should give continuity of help and that they themselves should be aware of the range of services which can be called upon. If volunteers are to be used to the best advantage they must be carefully and thoughtfully deployed by one who takes into account their special abilities, knowledge and aptitudes.

VOLUNTARY–STATUTORY CO-OPERATION

The value of co-operation between statutory and voluntary bodies is fully recognised by the Government. Several Ministerial circulars issued during recent years have asked local health and welfare authorities and housing authorities to establish and maintain close links with voluntary bodies working for old people, and to use all available means to encourage 'the expansion of voluntary effort along whatever lines have proved most fruitful'. In this connection local authorities have permissive powers to make grants to any voluntary body which is giving 'advice, information, and other assistance' or working 'for the benefit of the area or its residents'. The question as to which bodies should be helped and the amount of help which should be given is left to the discretion of the individual local authorities. Some of the most practical ways in which local authorities help voluntary organisations working for old people, are by making contributions towards the cost of providing meals or recreation, by giving or lending furniture, vehicles or equipment, by permitting voluntary bodies to use local authority premises, and by making available the services of local authority staff connected with the premises. Some authorities provide floor space, clerical help, or other assistance in place of, or in addition to making a grant.

As local authority powers to help voluntary bodies in their areas are permissive and flexible and as the effectiveness of organisation of the various voluntary bodies differs considerably from one area to another, it follows that there is no consistent pattern of voluntary-statutory co-operation throughout the country. Some local authorities are more generous than others in aiding voluntary organisations; some voluntary organisations are more reluctant than others to apply for aid, in the mistaken belief that this might impair their voluntary status; in some areas local authorities give actual financial aid but no services in kind, in others the opposite is true.

These factors should be noted in any consideration of voluntary activity in this country. Generalisations have to be made; there are exceptions to every generalisation; the strength of voluntary organisations is their adaptability to circumstances, their pragmatism, and the fact that it is the volunteers themselves – people with special aptitudes and attitudes – who bring the organisations into existence and make them function.

SOME NATIONAL VOLUNTARY ORGANISATIONS WHO ARE PARTICULARLY CONCERNED TO HELP THE ELDERLY

NATIONAL OLD PEOPLE'S WELFARE COUNCIL

(*See* chapter One)

Function and Organisation: The National Old People's Welfare Council acts as headquarters for over 1,500 old people's welfare committees throughout the country. An old people's welfare committee is a key organisation in the care of the elderly and it aims to be independent, non-political and widely representative in its area. An effective committee brings into regular consultation representatives of statutory and voluntary bodies and other interested individuals to ensure that a closely knit network which covers all the essential needs of the elderly is established.

A regional committee, for example, has representation from regional offices of central government departments, regional hospital boards, and from voluntary organisations working on a regional basis, and links together representatives of county old people's welfare committees throughout the area. A county old people's welfare committee normally has representation from local old people's welfare committees and from the principal voluntary organisations operating in the county, together with representatives of statutory bodies and particularly of the county council. Local committees cover a borough, an urban or rural disrict, a group of parishes or even one village. These committees co-ordinate the various branches of national and independent local voluntary organisations and statutory bodies working in the area, as well as link together individuals with special knowledge and experience, who do not belong to any particular voluntary organisation and who are not connected with local government. County borough committees function in county borough areas with similar representation and functions as local committees.

Each committee is autonomous; the function of the National Old People's Welfare Council is not to exert direct control over them but to provide a central source which will give information and advice: and will, when necessary, act as spokesman for all those concerned in old people's welfare. At the same time the National Council aims to set high standards of work and to help committees to maintain a consistently satisfactory level of achievement through its training schemes, advisory service and its field officers. A good old people's welfare committee is involved in a diverse and ever increasing number of activities to help the elderly in its area; see section below, 'The Kinds of Help given by Voluntary Organisations'.

It is increasingly felt that 'Committee' is not an appropriate name and that 'Association' or 'Council' is more suitable. There is also a widespread feeling that 'Old People's Welfare' is not a good title and many committees are now using names such as 'Association for the Elderly'. For convenience the term 'Committee' will be used throughout this publication.

Finance and Administration of Old People's Welfare Committees: Each committee is advised to adopt a constitution which gives charitable status in law. This enables it to obtain concessions relating to income tax, rates and entertainment duties. The National Old People's Welfare Council has drawn up a model constitution which has been accepted by the Charity Commission and the Inland Revenue. Committees normally raise a large part of their funds from various voluntary fund raising efforts. In addition to this, permissive legislation allows all local authorities in England and Wales, except parish councils, to make grants to old people's welfare committees as voluntary organisations for help with meals and recreation services (*see above*).

To function effectively, an old people's welfare committee needs money from the very beginning – for everyday expenses, such as postage and telephone, sometimes for office rent, heating and so on. As the work of co-ordinating effort and providing information develops, it is increasingly valuable for a committee to have a central office open regularly and for this a nucleus of whole time paid and trained staff is very desirable. Many committees rely on the valuable voluntary services of a part-time officer but committees in heavily populated areas have increasingly felt the need for permanent salaried personnel in order to make the most effective use of volunteers. Salaried appointments are being increasingly made. Grants towards Committees' administrative costs are obtainable from local authorities under the Local Government Act, 1948, Section 136 as defined above.

THE BRITISH RED CROSS SOCIETY

During the last fifty years, the British Red Cross Society has shown special and increasing concern for old people and nowadays it helps the elderly in a great variety of ways. Nursing members provide auxiliary nursing help in old people's homes and similar establishments; they help under the supervision of district nurses to care for elderly people who are ill in their own homes. Members of the Red Cross visit sick, elderly people in hospital and often arrange picture library services and help to run trolley shops.

There are a number of Red Cross residential homes and some which give holidays to the infirm and disabled. Recently, the Red Cross has concentrated particularly on providing more places in short-stay homes for elderly people and in arranging transport for relatives to visit those elderly who are isolated in geriatric units far removed from their familiar surroundings. The Society has representation on the National Old People's Welfare Council and on local old people's welfare committees and participates in visiting schemes, running meals-on-wheels services etc.

WOMEN'S ROYAL VOLUNTARY SERVICE

WRVS in England, Scotland and Wales is active in the provision of voluntary services for the elderly. WRVS runs 110 all-day clubs where mid-day meals are provided and over 2,000 clubs which meet for tea in the afternoons, organises savings schemes and holidays, day outings and Christmas shopping. Library services serve both the clubs and homebound people. WRVS also runs clubs and trolley shops in welfare homes and geriatric hospitals.

For elderly people living alone who find it too much of an effort to cook and have no incentive to feed themselves properly, luncheon clubs are organised; for those who are housebound WRVS delivers hot midday meals to their homes – in 1967 over nine million Meals-on-Wheels were being delivered in 1,800 areas and the scheme is continually being expanded. Many visiting services which ensure continuity of visiting are being run by WRVS; families, youth clubs and groups of school children, as well as individuals, take part. These visiting services often include help with shopping, letter writing, collecting pensions, gardening and house decorating.

WRVS runs twenty-three residential clubs for elderly people and two nursing homes where they can go if they are taken ill and need nursing care. During 1967 a new residential club was opened for old people not sufficiently able-bodied to live in a residential club, but not in need of skilled nursing.

The WRVS Housing Association co-operates in practical schemes to house elderly people on local authority housing lists and has been responsible for the erection and conversion of buildings where retired professional people can live at a rent which they can afford. WRVS is a constituent member of the National Old People's Welfare Council and has membership on county and local old people's welfare committees.

YOUTH GROUPS

In the last few years, young people who help the elderly have received an increasing amount of recognition and encouragement from the general public. The young people may belong to various church groups, to youth clubs, or to bodies such as Girl Guides, Boy Scouts or Red Cross cadets; they may be school children or students whose impetus to help comes from their teachers; they may be members of youth organisations specially formed to help those in the community with particular needs. Examples of the latter organisations are Task Force in the London area, the Youth Activities Movement in Portsmouth and Birmingham Young Volunteers' Trust. The establishment of the Young Volunteer Force Foundation, a new national body with government financial support, has just been announced. There are a great number of practical ways in which the young can help the elderly and many other ways – not necessarily so practical but equally valuable – in which the elderly can help the young.

CHURCH GROUPS

Nearly all religious denominations show a particular concern in one way or another for their elderly members. The Jewish community is helped in a number of ways by the Jewish Welfare Board and some churches, for example, the Catholic, the Methodist, the Society of Friends and the Church Army, run homes for the aged. Some, the Anglicans and Baptists for instance, provide homes for their own clergy and their dependants.

Church groups often co-operate with old people's welfare committees in visiting the elderly and some residential homes and clubs are regularly visited by local clergy of different denominations and services may be arranged. Nevertheless, it is felt that the spiritual needs of the elderly are not always adequately catered for, particularly those of the housebound. Therefore in 1967 the National Old People's Welfare Council arranged a preliminary consultation of members of religious bodies to discuss their role in connection with the care of the elderly. Meetings are to be held to consider ways in which the various religious groups can co-operate more effectively in looking after the needs of older people.

CITIZENS' ADVICE BUREAUX

Citizens' advice bureaux are able to give expert advice to elderly people on many subjects which are of immediate concern to them, for example rent, rates and tenancy problems; financial and legal affairs, etc. In areas where there is a bureau and an old people's welfare committee it is desirable to have representation on each other's committee so that close contact can be maintained. CAB workers sometimes visit outlying old people's clubs regularly so that the members can consult them without having to make a long journey to the office of the bureau.

KINDS OF HELP GIVEN BY VOLUNTARY ORGANISATIONS TO ASSIST THE ELDERLY

VISITING

The objects of a Visiting Service: In the changed pattern of our mobile society there are more elderly people who are either without relatives or who live alone long distances from them. As a result, an increasing number of older people tend to become isolated from the main stream of the community because they lack younger contacts with it; they see few people; often they know little about what can be done to help them. Naturally, some elderly people are quite content in a state of social isolation, but others suffer a sense of loneliness and deprivation and depression which may be accentuated by the death of a spouse or a dear friend. It is these elderly people whom a visiting service tries to help by bringing to them companionship, a sense of security and a sense of still belonging to a community that cares.

Organisation of a Visiting Service: Because it is a co-ordinating body, bringing together all those in an area interested in old people's welfare, the old people's welfare committee is very well suited to establishing a visiting service. In order to be effective, such a service needs to be run by a visiting organiser. The organiser sometimes works voluntarily; in other cases, the salary is paid by a local trust or the organiser receives a honorarium from the old people's welfare committee and, where a service is established, a grant towards administrative expenses may be made by local authorities. The latter arrangement is becoming more common in densely populated areas where a full-time organiser is needed. A visiting organiser helps in the recruiting, selecting and briefing of volunteers, the keeping of simple records, and the training of new volunteers. He or she ensures that visitors are aware of the services, both voluntary and statutory, which are available to the elderly, and all ways in which the lives of old people can be enriched through the development of new interests and affiliations. A visiting organiser also tries to maintain and increase the network of contacts between various voluntary organisations involved, so that the scope of the service can be enlarged and improved.

What visitors can do: Visitors can be male or female, young, middle-aged or fairly elderly themselves, drawn from all sections of the community. The main common denominator among those they visit is that they are old, tending to be isolated, housebound or semi-housebound. There are elderly people drawn from all walks of life and varieties of background who may need a visitor. The retired professional person can be as lonely as the ex-manual worker. Within the visiting pattern there are a great number of different roles which the visitors can perform according to their capacities and temperament, and that of the old people being visited. In some cases a visitor just sits and chats with the old person bringing news of the neighbourhood, and encouraging interest in the outside world. It is also part of a visitor's function to make sure that the old person has the full benefit of domiciliary services available, such as a home help, chiropody, and meals services where necessary. In addition the visitor often gives valuable personal service, bringing library books and magazines, collecting pensions, shopping, writing letters, reading aloud, and arranging outings for the old person to (say) a club, theatre, church or cinema. Visitors may help by sitting in with the old person while relatives go out, by playing cards with them, cooking the odd meal, bringing together old friends – in short finding out what in particular the old person needs and likes and trying to provide it.

It is sometimes forgotten too how much visits are appreciated by many who live in homes, housing schemes, hospitals or hotels. Even if there are not so many material and practical needs to cater for, the principle of visiting remains the same – elderly residents enjoy a personal relationship, a chat and an exchange of experience. Long-stay patients in geriatric wards are especially grateful for any visits or outings which help them to feel less cut off from the community as a whole.

It is very desirable that all types of friendly visiting should be carried on regularly so that an old person can rely on and look forward to the visitor's call. With regard to visitors to the old person's own home, there is often a special need for volunteers who are able to help with jobs around the house. Young people are of great value here; they help with gardening, cleaning a room, taking a dog for a walk, repairing a radio, clearing snow away, ironing, chopping wood and so on.

In addition to these planned visits of course, a neighbour often pops in to keep an eye on an old person, as do members of (say) the nearby club or church. Ideally, visitors complement each other's work and an old people's welfare committee can arrange this so that overlapping is avoided. Many clubs regularly visit their members who become sick or housebound and this should form part of the overall visiting service.

MOBILE MEALS

Mobile meals services are run in close conjunction with welfare authorities, which now have powers to operate the services themselves if they wish, but in many cases give financial aid to voluntary organisations which act as their agents or help with the provision of meals services. Local authorities generally have power to give grant aid for meals services and it can take the form of a contribution towards the provision of equipment and vehicles, wages and distribution costs; in some cases local authority staff, such as cooks and drivers, are employed, or the local authority offers garage accommodation for vans and help with maintenance. The recipients of meals pay a small charge which may cover the full cost of the meal or it may be subsidised from local authority or voluntary funds. The principal voluntary organisations which run meals services in this way on behalf of local authorities are Women's Royal Voluntary Service, old people's welfare committees, and the British Red Cross Society, often in co-operation with each other. The recipients are the aged, sick and disabled housebound, whose names are passed to the voluntary organisations either by their own visitors or by general practitioners, welfare officers, health visitors, district nurses, and so on.

Where the meals are prepared depends on what facilities are

locally available: kitchens belonging to the voluntary organisation concerned perhaps, a kitchen where school meals are prepared, kitchens of old people's homes, local restaurants or industrial canteens. The meals in special insulated containers are taken to recipients at mid-day either by vans or private cars. Keeping the meals hot is always a problem – slow combustion fuel drawers are used, electrical batteries, and experiments are now being made with micro-wave cooking appliances and with frozen foods. The number of meals which can be delivered depends on the size of area to be covered and the amount of money and staff available. Ideally, people who depend on mobile meals services for their main sustenance should receive them daily; but it is very difficult to maintain full services, particularly at weekends. Weekends are the time when the elderly housebound usually feel particularly lonely, so that provision of weekend meals is specially desirable. In this context, it should be stressed that the mobile meals service in general provides more than just a meal – it has definite social and psychological value because it gives the old person a sense of having someone to rely on, of being cared for, of belonging to the community. In addition, it affords a chance for the volunteer who delivers the meal to keep an eye on the old person regularly in case there is deterioration or some other welfare service is suddenly required.

(*For lunch clubs, see* chapter Eight.)

LAUNDRY SERVICE

In addition to the laundry services for the incontinent which are run by many local authorities (*see* chapter Three), a number of old people's welfare committees supplement these by the provision of a service for those who are not incontinent but because of frailty find it difficult to undertake their own laundering. Where this happens financial help is sometimes given by the local authority. Often the committee will have an arrangement with a local laundrette which allows old people to wash their linen at reduced rates during off-peak periods. In a few cases, old people's welfare committees or clubs have premises available of their own where they install washing machines and driers and sometimes operate a collection and delivery service. Occasionally the laundry services of hospitals or old people's homes provide facilities for old people's laundry.

CHIROPODY

This service, which was pioneered in the past by old people's welfare committees, has since 1959 become a recognised local authority responsibility (*see* chapter Three). Nevertheless, the voluntary – statutory pattern is still a varied one and in some areas a voluntary chiropody service is still carried on, sometimes because the local authority has failed to provide one, but more generally by mutual agreement between the committee and the authority concerned. Where voluntary organisations still perform this service, local authorities are empowered to give grants to help them in its administration and to pay the salary of a chiropodist. Local authorities may only employ qualified chiropodists, registered under the Professions Supplementary to Medicines Act, 1960, in their own services. They may, however, give grants to voluntary organisations employing qualified but non-registered chiropodists provided that the medical officer of health is satisfied that a reasonable standard of service is provided. Small charges may be made for chiropody treatment though some services – either by the local authority or a voluntary body – are made free to retirement pensioners.

Old people's welfare committees and the British Red Cross Society have been the most active voluntary organisations in this field and a particularly valuable contribution they have made has been to arrange, where possible, for chiropodists to give treatment to housebound old people in their own homes. Although they still contribute a great deal to the maintenance of chiropody services, voluntary organisations feel that chiropody is now most definitely a local authority responsibility and that they should not be expected to provide funds for it or to undertake detailed administrative work in connection with services.

NIGHT ATTENDANCE

The night attendance service provided by a voluntary body means that someone remains in the house of an old person at night, simply for companionship and to be on call in case of an emergency; she is not expected to provide any special nursing care. Such provision often makes it possible for old people to remain longer in their own homes instead of going to hospital or a residential home. It is therefore a very valuable form of help and one which needs expansion of both statutory and voluntary effort. An increasing number of local authorities provide some sort of night attendance service on a paid basis where trained nurses may be used (*see* chapter Three), but voluntary organisations concerned appear to be solely responsible in some areas and to augment local authority provision in others.

NURSING AIDS

Medical loan depots exist in most areas run by the British Red Cross Society, St John Ambulance Brigade and the local health authority to help those who are nursing the sick at home. Such items as wheel chairs, air-beds, bed-pans, and feeding spoons can be borrowed for as long as required; charges made, if any, are small.

DAY CENTRES AND CLUBS

(*See* chapter Eight.)

REFERENCES

Circulars and other HMSO Publications:

Local Government Act, 1948. HMSO, 7s 6d

National Assistance Act, 1948. HMSO, 5s 6d

National Assistance Act, 1948. (Amendment) Act, 1962. HMSO, 6d

Development of Local Authority Health and Welfare Services: Co-operation with Voluntary Organisations. Ministry of Health Circular 7/62, *Free*

Development of Local Authority Health and Welfare Services: Co-operation with Voluntary Organisations. Ministry of Health Circular 18/62, *Free*

Services for Old People. Joint Circular. Ministry of Housing and Local Government Circular 10/61, Ministry of Health Circular 12/61, 6d & 3d

Development of Local Authority Health and Welfare Services: Co-operation with Voluntary Bodies. Scottish Home and Health Department Circular 66/63, *Free*

Voluntary Effort in the Health and Welfare Services. Ministry of Health Circular 18/64, *Free*

For further reading:

(*A*) NOPWC/NCSS *Publications:*

Voluntary Visiting. A Manual for those Organising this Service for Old People. 1966, 2s 6d

Home Care of Old People. Pamphlet. 1963, 2d

Day Care Service for the Aged and Infirm in Their Own Homes. 1963, 2s 0d

Old People's Welfare Committees—Why they are needed: how they are started: what they do. 1965, 1s 3d

Looking After Old People At Home, D. Norton. 1962, 2s 6d

Youth Helps Age. 1964, 6d

(*B*) *Other Relevant Publications:*

Young People and Voluntary Service. NCSS, 1965, 2s 0d

The Caring Community. NCSS, 1968, 3s 0d

Voluntary Social Services. NCSS, 1965, 12s 6d (1967 Supplement 6d)

Loneliness. NCSS, 1964, 5s 6d

Voluntary Organisations and Social Progress, M. Morris. 1955, Victor Gollancz, 18s 0d

Lend A Hand, P. Campbell. 1965, Museum Press, 12s 6d

Outlines of a Survey on the Meals on Wheels Service. Summary of a report by the Government Social Survey. 1960, National Corporation for the Care of Old People, 2s 6d

Tragedies of Affluence. Salvation Army Centenary Booklet. 1965, 3s 6d

The Elderly Housebound, D. Snellgrove. 1963, White Crescent Press, Luton, 10s 0d

Useful Addresses:

British Red Cross Society,
12 Grosvenor Crescent, London SW 1

St John Ambulance Brigade,
8 Grosvenor Crescent, London SW 1

Women's Royal Voluntary Service,
17 Old Park Lane, London W 1

National Federation of Old Age Pensions Associations,
91 Preston New Road, Blackburn, Lancs

Salvation Army,
101 Queen Victoria Street, London EC 4

National Corporation for the Care of Old People,
Nuffield Lodge, Regent's Park, London NW 1

Help the Aged,
139 Oxford Street, London W 1

Royal National Institute for the Deaf,
105 Gower Street, London WC 1

Royal National Institute for the Blind,
224 Great Portland Street, London W 1

National Association for Mental Health,
39 Queen Anne Street, London W 1

Central Council for the Disabled,
34 Eccleston Square, London SW 1

National Council of Social Service,
26 Bedford Square, London WC 1
(for all local CSS and RCC addresses)

National Citizens' Advice Bureaux Council,
26 Bedford Square, London WC 1
(for all local CAB addresses)

CHAPTER FIVE

Accommodation

INTRODUCTORY

THE HISTORICAL BACKGROUND

The almshouses of the Middle Ages were the first attempt in Britain to provide permanent accommodation for the infirm aged. Many of the first almshouses were established and maintained by various religious orders; later, others were supported by groups of enlightened citizens (often belonging to the same trade or locality), or through the private generosity of a benefactor. The parish poor-houses and workhouses established during the seventeenth century housed many of the aged, often in miserable conditions. It was partly to offer more satisfactory alternative accommodation for certain groups – such as those who shared a religious belief or former occupation – that there was a great increase in the number of benevolent funds and trusts, many of which provided almshouse-type accommodation during the late eighteenth and nineteenth centuries.

Early in the twentieth century voluntary effort again paved the way for later state provision by the founding of small communal homes for those aged who needed nursing care. The Catholic and Anglican Sisterhoods, the Salvation Army and the Church Army were all pioneers in this field.

Before the second world war local authorities had built 48,800 houses for old people; and apart from this provided only communal accommodation for them chiefly in the wards of workhouse buildings which were, to say the least, cheerless places.

The hardships and deprivations that many old people suffered became increasingly apparent during the war years, and the formation of the National Old People's Welfare Committee in 1940 helped to bring this urgent matter to the public's attention.

RECENT DEVELOPMENTS

Since the 1940s considerable attention has been given to the planning and development of accommodation for old people both by statutory and voluntary bodies. The following are some of the main trends and principles which have emerged in recent years:

(1) It is now generally recognised that the majority of old people can and should, if they wish, live out their lives in their own homes surrounded by their own possessions.

(2) Some old people will be most comfortable if they remain in the home in which they have spent their working years; for others a move is desirable in order to provide the elderly with some conveniences, a smaller housing unit to manage or a more accessible location where they can keep in touch with the neighbouring community.

(3) There is an obvious need to design special accommodation for older people which will take into account their increasing disabilities and frailties while still enabling them to manage independently. In designing housing for the elderly certain general considerations should be borne in mind. Houses and flats need to be well insulated and equipped with effective, easily manageable heating systems; ergonomic considerations should be observed when installing cupboards, sink units, lighting and so on; doors may sometimes need to be wider to allow the passage of wheel chairs; aids, such as hand rails by the bath, need to be fitted; unnecessary steps should be avoided, and stairs should be shallow and wide with handrails.

(4) Many elderly people prefer and need small easily managed bungalows or flats. Nevertheless elderly people should be given the opportunity to choose where and how they will live and who they will live among. There is need for a greater variety of types of housing so that the old person can decide what is best for himself or herself.

(5) It is now accepted that when elderly people are no longer able to maintain an independent life in their homes and require care and attention in a residential home, they should live in small homes, and that the old workhouses should be abolished.

Since the war local authorities alone have provided 1,764 small homes for the elderly of which 724 were purpose-built. At the same time the numbers of old workhouses have been steadily reduced.

THE TYPES OF HOUSING AVAILABLE

INDEPENDENT OWNER OCCUPIED HOUSING

It is difficult for elderly people to obtain a loan from a local authority, building society or insurance company to buy a house. This depends on individual circumstances, however, and it is always worth making an approach. It is advisable for any buyer to seek professional advice before actually signing a contract of house purchase.

GROUPED ACCOMMODATION

Introductory: A large amount of the accommodation which has been specially built or converted for use by the elderly is in groups. It is obviously easier to provide supervision and care if old people's dwellings are grouped together. On the other hand, it is most important that the elderly should not be segregated and cut off from the everyday life of younger people. The National Old People's Welfare Council feels it is essential, in fact, that a balanced allocation of older and younger people in a community should be maintained as far as is practicable. When siting these dwellings it is also very important that there should be easy access to communal facilities such as public transport, libraries, shops, churches and public houses. This helps to alleviate some old people's feelings of social isolation.

The main types of grouped accommodation are: Converted houses with flatlets for six to twelve occupants; purpose-built groups of bungalows or blocks of flats which accommodate tenants in single or double units. In some cases grouped housing includes certain communal amenities such as a common room, guest room, laundry room. In the case of flatlets or bed-sitting rooms shared bathrooms are sometimes installed.

Warden Service: In increasing numbers of local authority and voluntary housing association grouped schemes for the elderly the provision of a warden service is included. Ideally, the job of a resident warden is to allow tenants to have the maximum amount of independence in their homes, and at the same time to be able to give security and support when required. It is not the warden's task either to supervise unduly the daily living of the tenants or to undertake extensive care of the sick. In any warden service scheme the warden is not a substitute for other domiciliary help or for the attention of relatives and friends. Her job is to supplement these, and to be available to deal with emergencies if necessary.

At present there is great diversity in the kinds of housing scheme where wardens are employed, the sort of duties they are expected to perform and their conditions of service. These are considered more fully in *Wardens and Old People's Dwellings* published by the National Old People's Welfare Council, 1966. Details of Training Courses for Wardens appear in chapter Six.

STATUTORY AND VOLUNTARY BODIES CONCERNED WITH HOUSING THE ELDERLY

LOCAL AUTHORITY HOUSING

In recent years about a quarter of the dwellings built by local authorities have been one-bedroom bungalows or flats suitable for old people. Nevertheless, there is still a nation-wide shortage of this kind of accommodation. Elderly people who want to move or think they may wish to do so in the future because their present accommodation is no longer suitable or convenient, should be advised to apply for admission to local authority housing lists. An applicant is more likely to be given a place on such a list if he has residential qualifications through living in the area for some time. However, present policy stresses that local authority housing should be allocated primarily on the basis of greatest need.

In comparison with current building costs, rents for local authority houses are low. Local authorities have sole responsibility for the management, regulation and control of the houses they own and may fix rents at any levels they consider reasonable. They may also grant rent rebates.

HOUSING ASSOCIATIONS

The National Federation of Housing Societies. In 1935 this co-ordinating 'central association' for the promotion and guidance of housing associations was established and reorganised under the Housing Acts. Housing associations are voluntary, non-profit making bodies which supplement the efforts of local authorities and private enterprise in the housing field. They provide accommodation to let (at as reasonable rents as possible) by new building with subsidy, and by conversion with improvement grants and special subsidy arrangements. As at November 1967, the membership of the National Federation of Housing Societies stands at over 1,600 affiliated housing associations and societies; of these some five hundred were formed with the specific aim of providing accommodation for old people. Many of the associations in this category have been established as a result of the efforts of voluntary workers – members of old people's welfare committees, Rotarians, church groups, for instance – in order to meet a particular local need. Such associations aim to help those elderly who, for example, do not qualify for a council tenancy, those who are living in large, isolated and inconvenient houses which they cannot afford to keep in good repair, or those who need the support of voluntary societies if they are to move to more suitable housing.

Other Housing Associations: In addition to housing associations which work primarily with the National Federation of Housing Societies, there are others which, while linked with the Federation, have been formed by other national bodies. There is, for example, the Hanover Housing Association, set up by the National Corporation for the Care of Old People, which operates on a national basis, as well as Mutual Households and the Soroptomists amongst others. There is also the Abbeyfield Society, which provides accommodation with meals for elderly people in individual houses, each taking five to seven tenants. Organisations of this kind all concentrate on providing small comfortable living units for elderly people, often with a resident housekeeper and at as reasonable a cost as possible.

Finance: Local authorities have permissive powers to assist housing associations in their areas by helping in the acquisition of suitable building land, by lending money towards capital expenditure on security of mortgage, by passing on to them certain Exchequer grants and subsidies, and by supplementing these grants from their own funds. In order to be eligible for such assistance, a housing association must fulfil certain conditions; in addition, most associations obtain legal status by registering under the Industrial and Provident Societies Act. In cases where housing projects, either new ones or conversions, include a welfare element specially for old people – such as accommodation for a resident warden – welfare grants from a county council or county borough council may be obtainable. In addition, the charitable type of housing association aiming to provide accommodation for the elderly obtain funds from donations, legacies and fund raising schemes; certain charitable trusts acting through the National Federation also make financial contributions to housing associations in some cases.

Under section 15 of the Housing Subsidies Act, 1967, an increased hostel grant is available to housing associations, such as the Abbeyfield Society, which provide some or all meals in addition to accommodation.

THE HOUSING CORPORATION

The Housing Corporation was set up under the Housing Act, 1964, to promote and assist the development of housing societies; in 1965, the Ministry of Housing and Local Government asked local authorities to encourage the development of these societies in the hope that eventually they would be operating in every sizeable town. These societies are established either on a cost rent or a co-ownership basis. A cost rent society is one which acts as a non-profit making landlord by charging rents which are not greater than is needed to cover outgoings. A co-ownership society provides accommodation which is occupied exclusively by its own members who collectively own the dwellings they occupy individually. Both these types of society are of interest to older people; a cost rent society because it aims to provide individual accommodation at a reasonable rent; a co-ownership society because it offers security of tenure to those who wish to live in their own houses but who perhaps find it difficult to raise sufficient capital to purchase one. Housing societies aim to raise about two-thirds of their capital outlay from building societies or other finance agencies; the rest is made up in loans from the Housing Corporation.

OTHER ORGANISATIONS PROVIDING ACCOMMODATION

Almshouses: The National Association of Almshouses is concerned with supporting and modernising existing almshouses, and in building new ones. The Association estimates that in 1966 there were about 2,500 almshouse foundations in Great Britain and that these provide accommodation for about 50,000 old people. Almshouses are traditionally groups of small dwellings or flatlets in which old people can live in relative independence, sometimes with the support of a warden. Capital grants for the repair and restoration of almshouses of outstanding architectural or historical importance are made by the Ministry of Housing and Local Government (on the recommendation of the Historic Buildings Council for England) and by the Pilgrim Trust, and the normal improvement grants are available.

Grants for other almshouses are sometimes obtainable from charitable trusts. In addition grants towards the cost of welfare services in almshouses might be obtainable from local welfare authorities. There is no up-to-date central register of vacancies available in almshouses and conditions of entry vary considerably. Details can be obtained direct from the Clerk of the Almshouses concerned.

Religious Denominations: Church Army Housing Ltd operate some sixty-seven Churchill Houses in various parts of the country. These houses contain one-room flatlets with built-in kitchen unit and are for those elderly people who can look after themselves; however, a housemother is in attendance to cope with emergencies.

Applications for entry should be made in the first instance to Church Army Housing Ltd.

One or two other religious denominations provide accommodation for some of their elderly members. This is usually in the form of flatlets or bed-sitting rooms in converted houses and is established on an individual and local scale according to need. Organisations doing this include the Society of Friends, Catholic Women's League and the Jewish Welfare Board.

FINANCIAL PROVISIONS FOR HOUSING

IMPROVEMENT GRANTS

For those who already own a house but one which needs modernisation, two kinds of grants are available from local authorities provided certain conditions are met: discretionary and standard improvement grants. The purpose of these grants is to finance improvements to property; it is not for repairs or for the renewal of obsolete or worn-out installation or equipment. The first objective is to provide amenities in houses that are structurally sound; the second is to increase the number of living units by converting large older houses into two or more flats or by bringing other buildings into housing use. Standard grants are given towards the provision of amenities such as bath, lavatory, hot and cold water supply. Discretionary grants are at the discretion of the local authority to help owners with more extensive improvements. Under certain circumstances a discretionary grant may be given towards the central heating of a dwelling which is specifically designed to house old people. Local authorities also have power to make loans under the Housing Acts for the conversion, improvement, repair and alteration of houses. Details of how to apply for either of the grants or for a loan are obtainable from the local council offices.

RENT REBATES IN LOCAL AUTHORITY HOUSING

About 44 per cent of the housing authorities in England and Wales operate a rent rebate scheme. The terms and conditions under which rent rebates are allowed differ from one local authority to another and application for rebate must be made to the particular local authority concerned.

PRIVATE RENTED ACCOMMODATION

Accommodation of this kind includes ordinary private houses, flats, bungalows or bed-sitting rooms. The Rent Act which came into effect in December 1965 aims to give security of tenure to tenants and to fix fair rents. Fair rents are defined as being those which would be fair for a house if there was no shortage of similar accommodation in the area, and they can be fixed for most unfurnished lettings where the rents are not controlled under the Rent Acts. A tenant who thinks his rent is too high can apply to the rent officer whose address may be obtained from the council offices. The rent officer will fix a rent and if either the landlord or the tenant object the rent officer will refer the matter to the Rent Assessment Committee. Where the accommodation is furnished, rent tribunals have power to fix rents in certain cases and may grant security of tenure for periods of up to six months. The address of the tribunal can be obtained from the council offices. Under the Rent Act, 1965, it is unlawful to evict a tenant without first obtaining an order from the Court.

In the case of the death of a married man who is the statutory tenant the right of tenancy passes to his widow or, where there is none, to any member of his family who has been residing with him for at least six months prior to his death. Such a tenancy can be transmitted twice, for example to the widow and subsequently to her son or daughter.

RATE REBATES

Under the Rating Act 1966 about two million rate payers in England and Wales who are living on low incomes can qualify for a substantial reduction in rates. Those who can apply for the rebate include owner-occupiers of houses and flats, tenants of private houses and tenants of council accommodation. At present a low income is defined as £8 or below for a single person; £10 a week or below for a couple. A person's total income is defined as including pensions and supplementary benefits but any capital he has is disregarded. Application for a rate rebate should be made to the rating authority not earlier than two months before the beginning and not later than the end of the rebate period to which it relates.

BOARDING-OUT SCHEMES

GENERAL

In an attempt to alleviate the grave shortage of accommodation for old people, especially for those who do not have a settled home of their own in a particular locality, a few areas have established boarding-out schemes. These schemes, by which an elderly man or woman is boarded in a private household are usually organised, at least partially, by local old people's welfare committees.

The schemes are not all of the same type: some make arrangements for long term stay, others for short stay; one old people's welfare committee has managed to place individual old people with each other for companionship; another specialises in boarding-out old people directly they come out of hospital. If any type of scheme is to be successful it must be organised in co-operation with other bodies such as the Ministry of Social Security (with regard to payment of weekly boarding charges where an old person has no source of income other than a retirement pension); with the various local authority and voluntary domiciliary services, such as home helps and meals services, and with interested individuals such as general practitioners, geriatric social workers and voluntary visitors.

THE BOARDING-OUT OFFICER

In order for a boarding-out scheme to operate efficiently it is essential that a paid boarding-out officer, preferably full time, should be appointed. The work of such an officer, who should have at least some knowledge of social case work, should be to establish and maintain contact with the various statutory and voluntary bodies concerned, to interview the elderly person and the householder offering accommodation and to keep in touch by means of follow-up visits to see that the arrangement is working satisfactorily. Local authorities have permissive powers to give financial aid to voluntary organisations towards the salary of the boarding-out officer and for other administrative expenses incurred in running such a scheme. Some local authorities already do this; in other cases committees have received initial assistance from trusts. Most old people's welfare committees establishing a boarding-out scheme must, however, be prepared to finance it partly, or even wholly, in its early stages until it has proved its worth.

RESIDENTIAL HOMES

There are three kinds of residential homes: local authority homes, homes run by voluntary organisations and private homes. At the end of 1966 the total number of elderly people in residential accommodation provided either directly by local authorities or through arrangements with voluntary organisations was 91,915. This figure has steadily increased in each of the last five years. Elderly people admitted to homes can broadly be categorised as those who, after careful assessment of their medical and social needs, cannot be expected to maintain themselves in their own homes. To perform its function satisfactorily a residential home should be designed and equipped to care for otherwise active residents during minor short-term illnesses, for the infirm who may need help with dressing etc, and who may spend longer periods in bed, and for those who have terminal illnesses and are not expected to live for more than a few weeks.

LOCAL AUTHORITY HOMES

Present position: In 1948 the National Assistance Act placed a duty on county and county borough councils to provide residential accommodation for persons who 'by reason of age, infirmity or any other circumstances are in need of care and attention which is not otherwise available to them'. Since 1st April 1965, a similar duty has been placed on London borough councils. The authority to provide such accommodation should be the one in whose area the person is normally resident. The term 'residential accommodation' includes not only provision of food and lodging but of social and recreational opportunities and generally comfortable living conditions. To achieve this local authorities are asked by the Ministry of Health to ensure that staffing of each home is sufficient to provide proper care for each resident and that as full a range of health and welfare services is available to residents as would be if they were living in good circumstances in their own homes. These are intended to include such services as chiropody, home nursing and the attention of a personal doctor when necessary.

During 1966, 128 new homes for the elderly were opened in England and Wales with accommodation for 5,777 residents. Of these 119 were new purpose-built buildings generally accommodating between thirty to fifty persons. Present policy favours such homes rather than the adaptation of existing premises. The number of old public institutions is also decreasing (ten were closed in 1966); nevertheless about 24,000 persons including some 21,500 elderly still live in former institutions or in joint-user premises shared with hospitals.

Financial Arrangements: Residents pay for the care they receive at a standard rate which is fixed by the local authority that maintains the home in which they live. A person who satisfies the authority that he is not able to pay the standard rate is assessed at a lower rate which must not fall below a minimum laid down by the Ministry of Health.

This minimum must still leave an individual a fixed sum of money, also specified by the Ministry, to meet his personal requirements. Those residing in local authority homes who do not have sufficient money to pay the minimum charge and have the sum specified for personal expenses are entitled to a supplementary pension or allowance from the Ministry of Social Security.

VOLUNTARY AND PRIVATE HOMES

Present position: A voluntary home is one which is owned by a non-profit-making body, usually a charity; a private home is one which is run for profit, usually by an individual or a limited company. While voluntary organisations were instrumental in the pioneering of residential homes, the number of voluntary homes is not nowadays increasing as rapidly as that of local authority homes. In general, voluntary organisations realise that much as they might wish to provide accommodation for elderly residents in a particular area or for a special group in the community it is a very serious responsibility to undertake. The fact that residents will become increasingly infirm must be faced from the start, and present policy, which encourages the elderly to remain in their own dwellings for as long as possible, means that residents are usually fairly infirm when they are first admitted. Such elderly people need a great deal of personal care and only those voluntary organisations which are fully prepared to meet the resulting extensive commitments in terms of money and staff should be encouraged to embark upon such projects.

Local authorities are responsible for the registration and inspection of privately run and voluntary homes. Recently, details have been made available defining more exactly the standards required of voluntary and private homes in such matters as bed space, staff ratio and general provision of facilities. A local authority is empowered to limit the number of persons in a home according to the amenities available and to stipulate the extent of its services.

Financial arrangements: The National Assistance Act 1948 (Section 26) allows county, county borough and London borough councils to contribute by means of direct grant to those voluntary organisations (including housing associations) which already provide, or are proposing to provide, homes for old people. A number of authorities also maintain elderly persons in accommodation provided by voluntary organisations on their behalf. 11,057 persons were so maintained at the end of 1966. The authorities pay such fees as are agreed and themselves charge the residents on the same basis as would apply if they were in local authority homes.

GENERAL PRINCIPLES AND FUTURE TRENDS

Residents: Residents in a residential home are encouraged to maintain as many links as possible with their community. Consequently they should not be taken too far from their own neighbourhood – so that they can for instance attend the same church or club as formerly and keep in touch with the same friends. In this context too they need to be given facilities for entertaining their own visitors privately. Kitchenettes or coffee kitchens are admirable for this purpose, giving residents the opportunity to make tea or coffee to serve in their own rooms. Residents should not feel any sense of restraint about this and should feel equally free to pay visits and take holidays as far as their physical disabilities will allow.

The Staff: The whole question of the staffing of residential homes – conditions of service, duties, recruitment and methods of training – has been studied by the Williams Committee on the staffing of residential homes and its views and recommendations are published in the committee report *Caring for People.* It is sufficient here to state a few general principles contained in the report – that the staff of residential homes are entitled to expect:

(1) good residential accommodation for themselves and for any dependants they may have;
(2) salaries commensurate with their qualifications and experience;
(3) reasonable hours of work;
(4) explicit arrangements for superannuation payments and related benefits.

It is desirable for professional staff to encourage the visits of voluntary helpers to homes wherever possible. In some cases voluntary helpers may perform small services to relieve an overburdened staff; for example preparing and serving afternoon tea, checking laundry, arranging flowers etc. In other cases, probably the majority, a voluntary helper's most useful role is to enrich the social life of the residents. A helper who regularly comes to a home bringing news of the neighbourhood and stimulating residents to maintain interest in a variety of outside activities makes a very valuable contribution to the life of the home.

The Premises: At the time of preparing this publication the Ministry of Health is revising its Building Note. This document sets out the standards which the Ministry has laid down as a guide for local authorities when planning new homes. The National Old People's Welfare Council fully supports the view that single and double rooms (the latter for married couples or friends) should be provided which can be furnished by the residents themselves so that they create the feeling of an individual 'home' and not an impersonal bedroom in an institution. Adequate and convenient accommodation for residential staff is essential including where necessary provision for married couples. (*See: Residential Homes for the Elderly,* National Old People's Welfare Council.)

Homes for the Mentally Infirm: The Ministry of Health consider that in general elderly mentally infirm persons should be cared for individually or in small groups in ordinary residential homes for the elderly. They envisage, however, that specialised homes may be advisable in some circumstances for such persons who cannot be suitably accommodated in an ordinary home, particularly if the special home does not have too large a catchment area. Most needs, cannot be expected to maintain themselves in their own to continue to look after residents in ordinary homes who become a little mentally frail, provided they do not upset the other residents or become too great a burden on the staff. Local psychiatric services should be able to help in the care of such residents.

REFERENCES

Ministry Circulars and HMSO Publications:

More Flatlets for Old People. Ministry of Housing and Local Government, 1960, HMSO, 2s 0d

Flatlets for Old People. Ministry of Housing and Local Government, revised 1962, HMSO, 2s 6d

Some Aspects of Designing for Old People. Ministry of Housing and Local Government, 1962, HMSO, 2s 6d
Grouped Flatlets for Old People. Ministry of Housing and Local Government, 1962, HMSO, 5s 0d
Residential Accommodation for Elderly People. Local Authority Building Note no 2, 1962, HMSO, 2s 3d
Contributions to Voluntary Bodies. Ministry of Housing circular 43/64, HMSO, 3d
Flats for Disabled. Ministry of Housing circular 54/64, HMSO, 6d
House Improvement. Ministry of Housing circular 41/65, HMSO, 9d
The Rent Act and You. 1965, HMSO, 9d
Estimates, Expenditure, and Rates. Ministry of Housing and Local Government circular 29/66, Ministry of Housing, Whitehall, *Free*
Subsidies for Housing Associations. Housing Subsidies Act 1967—Part I. Ministry of Housing and Local Government, HMSO, 1s 6d
Residential Hostels for the Mentally Disordered. Local Authority Building Note no 6, 1967, HMSO, 2s 0d
Rates Rebates. Ministry of Housing and Local Government circular R.N.14, 1966, *Free*

For further reading:

(*A*) NOPWC/NCSS *Publications:*

Housing for the Elderly (Published jointly with the National Federation of Housing Societies). 1964, 2s 0d
Wardens and Old People's Dwellings. 1966, 9d
Boarding-Out Schemes for the Elderly. 1966, 1s 9d
Residential Homes for the Elderly (Evidence presented to the Williams Committee). 1966, 4s 0d

(*B*) *Other Relevant Publications:*

The Last Refuge, P. Townsend. 1964, Routledge and Kegan Paul, 30s 0d; Paperback edition 10s 6d
Housing Associations and Societies. National Federation of Housing Societies. 1966, 2s 6d
Buying a House or Flat – Do's and Dont's. Published for National Citizens Advice Bureaux Council, NCSS. 1967, 2s 6d
Peace at the Last, H. L. Glyn Hughes. 1960, Gulbenkian Foundation, 98 Portand Place, London W 1, 5s 0d
Nursing Homes in England and Wales, C. Woodroffe and P. Townsend. 1961, National Corporation for the Care of Old People, Nuffield Lodge, Regent's Park, London NW 1, 7s 6d
Accommodation for the Mentally Infirm Aged. 1963, National Corporation for the Care of Old People, 2s 6d
Institutional Neurosis, R. Barton. 1960, John Wright & Sons, Bristol, 8s 6d
Old People in Homes, P. Shaw. 1963, Faber & Faber, 18s 0d

Church Army Housing. Church Army Housing, (booklet) 1966, *Free Housing for Old People.* Programme Advisory Service leaflet no 25, 1961, Rotary International, 6d
Private Homes for Old People. 1967, National Corporation for the Care of Old People, 5s 0d
Caring for People. Staffing Residential Homes. Report of the Williams Committee. 1967, Allen and Unwin, 32s 0d
Annual Charities Digest. Family Welfare Association and Butterworth, 18s 6d
Problems of Accommodation and Medical Social Care of Old People. Council of Europe Committee of Experts on Public Health. Presented by Prof E. Aujaleu (France), Strasbourg 1965

Useful addresses:

National Federation of Housing Societies,
86 The Strand, London WC 2

Elderly Invalids Fund,
10 Fleet Street, London EC 2

WRVS Housing Association,
17 Old Park Lane, London W 1

Abbeyfield Society,
23 Nottingham Place, London W 1

Church Army Housing Ltd,
185 Marylebone Road, London NW 1

Salvation Army,
101 Queen Victoria Street, London EC 4

National Association of Almshouses,
Billingbear Lodge, Wokingham, Berks

Mutual Households Association Ltd,
41 Kingsway, London WC 2

Hanover Housing Association,
77 Church Road, Ashford, Middx

Methodist Homes for the Aged,
1 Central Buildings, Westminster, London SW 1

CHAPTER SIX

Training in the care of the elderly

PROVIDED BY THE NATIONAL OLD PEOPLE'S WELFARE COUNCIL

THE NEED FOR TRAINING

In the provision of a comprehensive and fully developed service for the elderly, volunteers always have, and as far as one can tell, always will have an essential part to play. If volunteers are to perform their work successfully and effectively they need an appropriate preparatory training. The aims of such training should be to make volunteers aware of the principal needs of the elderly, informed about the full range of services that exist, imaginative about possibilities of development and co-operative in relationships both with statutory authorities and other voluntary organisations. Training is needed to deepen insight, improve standards of work and strengthen the sense of responsibility. Volunteers thus equipped can be of immense help and comfort to elderly people in general, and in particular to the very old who are often bereft of close family ties and isolated from the community.

The emphasis nowadays is on helping elderly people to remain in their own homes as long as possible with the help of voluntary and statutory domiciliary services. Neverthcless there are a number who, because of increasing infirmity, can eventually be best cared for in a residential home, and in this field there is a continuing and urgent need to train wardens, matrons and assistant matrons so that they may be helped to carry out their responsible and demanding jobs with sympathy and imagination. Training is also necessary to help develop capabilities and give additional stimulus to those who are already working with the elderly in a professional capacity.

Social workers, wardens of housing projects, tutors who will in turn train others, all benefit from carefully planned relevant courses of instruction which help them to improve and expand their work.

KINDS OF TRAINING AVAILABLE

KING GEORGE VI SOCIAL SERVICE SCHEME

Establishment and Development: A grant of £40,000 was given to the National Old People's Welfare Council in 1954 by the King George VI Foundation to provide training for those engaged in the care and welfare of old people; such training to be primarily for voluntary workers, but to include some full time paid staff. The Social Service Scheme, as it became known, was a pioneer in the field because it made possible for the first time a systematic plan for short term training in the care of the elderly. The early scheme was so successful that after three years the Foundation increased the grant to £105,000 to enable the work to continue for a further period.

In its early stages the scheme was concerned principally with making the concept of training acceptable. In the second phase ideas of progression and continuity were developed. Experiments were made with different types and patterns of training adapted to local experience and with a view to improving quality. More recently particular stress has been put upon initiating and developing training schemes in co-operation with the Universities, statutory authorities and other bodies responsible for further education.

At the present time a small permanent residue from the King George VI Social Service Scheme Fund, augmented by a grant from the Sembal Trust, remains to provide advisory services and to support certain national courses, and a bursary fund, with a view to continued pioneer and experimental development. The aims, methods and standards of the scheme are formulated by the Training Committee of the National Old People's Welfare Council.

Each locality has been encouraged to prepare a systematic plan of training over a period. A number of education and welfare authorities make annual grants to old people's welfare committees which assist them to meet administrative and tutoring costs.

Courses for voluntary workers and staff of voluntary agencies

(1) *Nationally organised residential courses* for key workers, such as secretaries and other officers of old people's welfare committees, organisers of voluntary visiting schemes and of all-day clubs. Courses for the training of tutors are held from time to time, since it is important to train people who will in turn teach others.

(2) *Leaders' courses* (often residential) held in counties and cities to help key people to initiate and organise local courses; these have also been designed to assist overall planning of services.

(3) *Local courses* for groups of voluntary workers to help the elderly in various ways. Participants, brought together from a variety of organisations, include visitors, club workers, mobile meals helpers and new recruits.

(4) *Specialised courses* planned for particular groups which give one particular service, such as groups of visitors, of club leaders or youth helpers.

(5) *Day conferences* are organised nationally, regionally and locally; often these are concerned with a single issue, such as 'Youth in the Service of Age'.

Courses and Schemes for Paid Workers

(1) The King George VI Social Service Scheme has also pioneered a number of special courses for professional or experienced full time social workers employed by statutory or voluntary bodies, all or part of whose time is devoted to old people. These courses have had particular success in London.

(2) Courses for wardens of housing projects for the elderly were begun in 1962 on a residential national basis. They are now being provided by regional and county old people's welfare committees and by the local welfare and education authorities.

Training Methods and Curricula

(1) The provision of literature, teaching aids and other teaching material is an important part of the Social Service Scheme. Films, film strips, role plays, discussion group briefs and reading lists

are available from the National Old People's Welfare Council and this material is regularly supplemented and brought up to date.

(2) Curricula of national, leaders or local courses held for voluntary workers cover such subjects as: attitudes towards ageing, physical and mental health of the elderly, the work of old people's welfare committees, the scope of service available, techniques of visiting, club management.

(3) Curricula of specialised courses for voluntary and paid workers concentrate particularly on topics of immediate relevance to the service for the elderly with which the group is concerned.

PRELIMINARY COURSES FOR SECRETARIES AND OFFICERS OF OLD PEOPLE'S WELFARE COMMITTEES AND AWARD OF BURSARIES

Ideally, secretaries and organisers of voluntary associations for old people's welfare should have a *recognised training* in social work and some practical experience of social organisation.

Duties of secretaries/organisers include enlisting support of constituent bodies, making good use of existing services, recruiting new volunteers, providing advisory services to help elderly people who are in difficulty. To perform this task well the secretary/organiser must have a genuine wish to help the elderly; he/she also needs practical training in social and administrative techniques and to be well informed about the whole field of old people's welfare.

The National Old People's Welfare Council is at present able to offer a limited number of *bursaries* yearly of value up to £150 each, to enable newly-appointed secretaries of old people's welfare committees to take a preliminary course of practical work and study. Details of bursaries and periods of training are arranged according to the needs of individual applicants. There is also a training fund which makes grants of not more than £20 to enable officers of old people's welfare committees to attend short courses arranged by the National Old People's Welfare Council, or in co-operation with it.

TRAINING AND CO-OPERATION WITH UNIVERSITIES, STATUTORY AUTHORITIES AND ADULT EDUCATION BODIES

CO-OPERATION WITH UNIVERSITIES

The National Old People's Welfare Council has co-operated with extra-mural departments of universities to provide specialised courses for those engaged in a particular aspect of the work. In addition since 1965 an annual seminar has been held in conjunction with the University of Cambridge Board of Extra-Mural Studies. These seminars are for senior officers of statutory and voluntary bodies and deal with particular aspects of policy planning for the elderly population.

In recent years, LOCAL EDUCATION AUTHORITIES AND OTHER BODIES CONCERNED WITH ADULT EDUCATION have been accepting more responsibility for the training of voluntary workers in old people's welfare. As already mentioned, several authorities make annual grants to old people's welfare committees for support of their training programmes, and in many areas education departments and associated bodies offer facilities for courses, by making personnel available, providing premises and helping with administration. Where old people's welfare committees have not taken the initiative in training voluntary workers, statutory authorities are beginning to give a lead.

TRAINING FOR WARDENS, MATRONS AND ASSISTANT MATRONS OF HOMES

RECOMMENDATIONS OF THE WILLIAMS COMMITTEE

'Training for all forms of residential care is essential'. This is the conclusion of the Williams Committee and heads the recommendations on training in its report, *Caring for People,* published in May 1967. The Committee draws attention to the very great skills demanded of heads of residential homes and recommends a completely new pattern of training for the staff. This would provide a common basis of training for all those engaged in residential work, consisting of two-year courses with common subjects in the first year and specialisation in the second year. The four specialisations recommended are: children and young people; the elderly; the physically handicapped and the socially handicapped, and one or two of these subjects would be taken in conjunction with the main course. It is also suggested that for some older and experienced students there should be specialised one-year courses for a limited experimental period. A national training body would be needed to foster training developments, set standards and encourage research.

These recommendations overshadow any discussion of the training of staff of homes for the elderly, but as it is not known how soon or in what form they will be implemented, this chapter goes on to describe the existing training facilities which are available.

TRAINING PROVIDED BY THE NATIONAL OLD PEOPLE'S WELFARE COUNCIL

The need to provide some training to help the staff of residential homes was recognised early by the National Old People's Welfare Council, and the first refresher course for wardens and matrons was held in 1949, a year after the implementation of the National Assistance Act. In 1950 funds were made available by the National Corporation for the Care of Old People for the Council to pioneer a short training course for those wishing to become wardens, matrons and assistant matrons, and both types of courses are still in operation. Details of them are as follows:

Fourteen-week Training Courses: These courses are full-time, held twice a year and include both theoretical study and practical work, as follows: three weeks practical training in an old people's home; four weeks of theoretical training; four weeks in a hospital geriatric unit; three weeks in another old people's home; two days tuition at a residential centre. Subjects studied at the course include social background and legislation, human relationships, home management and catering, home nursing, the mental and physical aspects of ageing, occupational and social activities.

The courses are open to new recruits or to existing staff seeking promotion. As the present course is so short in relation to the skills and complexities of the work, some previous experience of residential or similar work is now considered to be highly desirable. The Council will assist in arranging preliminary experience for those who need it.

Grants are available to help with the cost of these courses. It is open to all students to apply to their local education authority for grant aid, and financial help may also be given through funds placed at the disposal of the National Old People's Welfare Council. For ten years from 1955 these courses were run with financial assistance from the King George VI Social Service Scheme and they are now again grant-aided by the National Corporation for the Care of Old People.

Refresher Courses and Special Emphasis Courses: These are residential courses, mostly of five days' duration, and are for wardens and matrons already in posts. They are also open to assistant wardens and matrons, and to a limited number of administrative officers and committee members. At refresher courses the programme is designed to cover a range of subjects related to the care of the elderly in homes, whereas at special emphasis courses one theme is taken and developed in greater depth.

Examples of subjects studied at refresher courses are: home management, personal and staff relationships, the care of the physically and mentally frail, catering, social activities and contacts with the neighbourhood. Themes taken at special emphasis courses have included: The matron and the staff, group and personal relationships, handicapped residents and how to help them.

At first both refresher and special emphasis courses were organised directly by the National Old People's Welfare Council and separate courses were organised by the Scottish Old People's Welfare Committee for wardens and matrons in Scotland. Recently local education authorities and residential colleges of adult education have provided some of the refresher courses in close collaboration with the National Old People's Welfare Council.

In-Service Training Provided by Local Authorities: A number of local health and welfare authorities have provided courses for their own staff or have combined with neighbouring authorities to do so. Sometimes these courses have been residential and sometimes on a day-release basis.

Day Conferences for wardens and matrons have been organised from time to time by regional and county old people's welfare committees. Conferences for members of committees responsible for the management of homes have also been organised by the National Old People's Welfare Council and the Scottish Old People's Welfare Committee. These conferences are invaluable in bringing together people in one neighbourhood or with a particular role in relation to residential care, but they are not intended as a substitute for longer and more comprehensive courses.

PRACTICAL WORK TRAINING FOR FULL-TIME SOCIAL SCIENCE STUDENTS

It is now realised that old people's welfare committees can offer a valuable opportunity to social science students interested in the welfare of the elderly to study aspects of and participate in a secretary's work, such as running a visiting service, attending committee meetings. Visiting clubs and day centres can be of great practical help to a student. Facilities for such training can only be offered where the old people's welfare staff is qualified to provide satisfactory guidance and where office space is adequate. The length of students' visits to old people's welfare committees vary from a one day tour of observation to block periods of six or eight weeks, or for two to three days a week for periods up to six months.

RESULTS OF TRAINING AND FUTURE PATTERNS

SOME RESULTS OF TRAINING

It is specially significant that statutory education authorities have begun to accept responsibility for the training of voluntary workers. A number of counties now give grants to old people's welfare committees for this purpose and local authority departments and educational bodies generally are helping with courses (*see above*). As yet, no planned research has been undertaken to find out whether improved standards of work have resulted from the courses given. Nevertheless, certain encouraging trends have developed in recent years which suggest that training in the care of the elderly is having a beneficial effect: They are as follows:

There is a more wide-spread knowledge of old people's needs and how to meet them, and a more thoughtful and sympathetic approach to the whole process of ageing.

New services have been started and existing ones revitalised.

Co-operation between voluntary and statutory workers in the field has become more fruitful. Voluntary workers are becoming more aware of the range of the statutory services available and how to use them; statutory workers are recognising the value of voluntary support.

Volunteers are realising the importance of planned expansion in their work and of developing an imaginative and responsible approach to it.

The standard and organisation of visiting services for the elderly have generally improved.

Courses for the staff of residential homes run by the National Old People's Welfare Council have helped in setting standards and providing a nucleus of suitably qualified personnel and proving the value and importance of well-planned training for this work. Refresher courses for staff have given valuable help in improving the quality of care received by residents and in broadening the horizons of those engaged in the work.

FUTURE PATTERNS IN TRAINING

Voluntary and Paid Workers caring for the Elderly: In view of the growing need for voluntary workers, the willingness of different kinds of people to serve, and the increasingly complicated patterns of our social services, it is essential to re-examine the question of effective training. Matters for future consideration include an assessment of suitable levels of training, its relationship to other kinds of social work, the wider aspects of community care and the further training of tutors. Greater exploration is needed into which agencies, including the universities, can help in the promotion of courses for voluntary workers. Future needs will be for a greater variety of courses at different levels, a greater emphasis than at present on preventive and constructive care in general and on certain specific and pressing problems – such as the care of the mentally frail living in their own homes.

The relationship of voluntary work to professional social work is a focus of growing interest, as was shown in the United Nations European Seminars held in 1966 and 1967 on the Functions and Training of Voluntary Social Welfare Workers. Professional social workers are increasingly concerned with the preparation and duties of volunteers and this is reflected in the appointment of the Aves Committee on Voluntary Workers in the Social Services, whose report will appear after the publication of this book.

Staff of Residential Homes: In considering the future, readers can do no better than study the report of the Williams Committee, to which reference has already been made. The staff of old people's homes need greatly extended training facilities so that they can develop their skills in personal relationships and practical care. The Williams Committee has a vision of residential care staff becoming ultimately a new professional group within the social services. Only a long-term scheme can make this possible.

REFERENCES

NOPWC/NCSS *Publications:*

The King George VI Social Service Scheme. Reprint of an article, 1966, *Free*

Training Courses for those engaged in welfare work among the elderly. Approaches for support to local authorities and other adult education bodies. *Free leaflet*

The function of old people's welfare committees in providing practical work training for students from social science departments of universities, colleges of further education, etc, and others preparing for social work as a profession. 1966, *Free leaflet*

Training courses for wardens, matrons and assistant matrons of old people's homes. *Free leaflet*

Residential Homes for the Elderly. Evidence to the Williams Committee. 1966, 4s 0d

Employment in the Care of the Elderly. Stencilled sheet, *Free*

A Manual of Voluntary Visiting for those organising this service for old people. 1967, 2s 6d

Youth Helps Age. 1964, 6d

Youth in the service of Age. 1966, 6d

Visual Aid Material concerned with the Care of the Elderly. List 6d

Other relevant publications:

The Field Training of Social Workers, S. Clement Brown and E. R. Gloyne. 1966, Allen and Unwin, paperback edition, 18s 0d

Lend A Hand, M. Campbell. 1965, Museum Press, 12s 6d

Adult Education. Year Book of the National Institute of Adult Education. 10s 0d

Caring for People. Staffing Residential Homes. Report of the Williams Committee. 1967, Allen and Unwin. 32s 0d

Educating older people, M. E. Cleugh. 1962, Tavistock Publications, 30s 0d

Training and Employment in Social Work. 1966, NCSS, 5s 0d

Field Work in Social Administration Courses. 1966, NCSS, published for the National Institute for Social Work Training, 6s 0d

Useful addresses:

National Institute for Social Work Training,
Mary Ward House, 5 Tavistock Place, London WC 1

Social Work Advisory Service,
26 Bloomsbury Way, London WC 1

Council for Training in Social Work,
Clifton House, Euston Road, London WC 1

National Institute for Adult Education,
35 Queen Anne Street, London W 1

CHAPTER SEVEN

Employment of the older worker

INTRODUCTORY

It is now commonly accepted that ageing is an individual process; people do not grow older at the same rate either biologically or psychologically; therefore they are not all ready to retire at the same point in their lives. The present widespread practice of compulsorily retiring men and women simply because they have reached the statutory retirement ages of sixty-five and sixty is a cause of anxiety and unhappiness among some elderly people.

Obviously there are many older people who are prepared for and look forward to their retirement and by exploring new enthusiasms, developing tried interests and participating in voluntary activities, they experience many enjoyable and fruitful retirement years. It is not suggested that elderly people should be persuaded to work longer than they wish to or indeed that they should feel in the least guilty about enjoying their well-earned leisure. However, retirement – for everybody – has two immediate impacts:

(1) the necessity of living on a pension as opposed to pay
(2) the sudden loss of the stimulus of work, the status or purpose that it gives, and the companionship it provides (and of which most people are unaware).

In addition, from a purely practical standpoint the fixing of an arbitrary age for retirement means that some are debarred from contributing several further years of productive work; it means that others who are less active and have aged earlier are forced to continue working, often with increasing inefficiency and absenteeism, beyond the limits of their physical stamina. Surveys carried out both in this country and other highly industrialised societies (where the statutory retiring age is not always the same as the British) show that in formulating their retirement policies employers in general think almost exclusively of the prevailing economic needs rather than the psychological and physical condition of the employee. That economic considerations are paramount is also suggested by the fact that in times of national crises, such as war, older people continue working successfully beyond the normal retirement age but in times of slump or oversupply on the labour market they are more or less forced to retire earlier. Studies of older workers reveal that their prime motive for continuing work is financial need, but many also state a preference for work in any case; the main reasons for leaving work are given as ill-health, lack of opportunity, compulsion by employer – in that order. While it is reasonable enough that economic factors and current supply of manpower must exert great influence in particular cases, this nevertheless should not rule out attempts to adopt a generally more flexible, humanitarian and far-sighted policy towards the whole question of compulsory retirement.

DEVELOPMENTS PAST AND PRESENT

GENERAL TRENDS

During the last fifteen years or so both government and industry have become aware that the present position concerning the older worker is not satisfactory having regard to the changing age structure in the population, the increasing life expectancy and future manpower needs. In 1953, 1954 and 1955 specially appointed Government Committees considered the question and made recommendations; in 1964 the National Corporation for the Care of Old People issued a report about the employment of the older woman. In recent years, too, several sociologists have looked at the problem and all have stressed the need for the formulation of a coherent policy on how the nation can best use and help its older workers.

(*For details of reports and publications see further reference section.*)

While it is evident that governments have in the past made only sporadic and piecemeal attempts to tackle the problem, voluntary organisations have for many years made considerable efforts to ensure that those elderly people who wish to continue in some kind of productive paid work should have the opportunity to do so. Recently, however, interest in the matter has become more widespread and the schemes and projects listed below are increasing their scope to meet a growing need.

VOLUNTARY EMPLOYMENT BUREAUX

General organisation: In order to help those elderly people who still wish to work, local organisations in some areas have set up voluntary employment bureaux and these are now operating in, for example, Cambridge, Luton, Stoke on Trent, Brighton, Oxford, Bradford, Stevenage and Slough. The bureaux usually operate for several hours on certain weekdays and are staffed by volunteers. The volunteers keep simple records of registration, interview older people seeking employment and aim to establish and maintain personal contact with employers in the area who are sympathetic and to persuade others of the worth and reliability of the older worker.

Finance and allied problems: Usually these bureaux are run in co-operation with and sometimes as part of the work of a local old people's welfare committee; in several cases office space and other help is given by the council of social service in the town. In one or two places some grant aid is given by local authorities towards the provision of office equipment and overhead expenses; in most cases the bureau has to rely almost entirely on voluntary funds though occasionally small registration fees are charged. Nearly all the bureaux are short of funds and often do not have enough office space or clerical help to enable them to expand their activities. As with most other forms of voluntary activities there is no overall pattern of development and each bureau is developed along individual lines according to the local employment situation, the attitude of employers and the personalities and influence of the volunteers concerned.

In addition to difficulties of finance common to all the bureaux, some have special problems. Naturally, for example, the kinds of job available depend to some extent on the local labour situation; in most areas the greatest demand from employers is for semi-skilled manual workers and those who will do gardening and domestic work. A majority of elderly people, however, seek white collar part-time jobs and it is very difficult to place professional men and women in the sort of work where they can continue to exercise their real abilities. Some elderly people who apply for work are limited by physical disability in what they can actually undertake: others are unwilling to take jobs of lower status or adapt their hours of work according to the employers' needs. Voluntary bureaux aim to maintain good relationships with local employment exchanges and in some cases Ministry of Labour officers send old people to the bureaux for help; in other areas, however, employment exchanges are not very sympathetic towards the bureaux' aims and feel that they themselves are doing everything necessary. In spite of these difficulties most voluntary bureaux have enlarged their scope and, once they are established, find that an increasing number of elderly people come to them seeking work.

WORK ROOMS FOR THE ELDERLY

The first work room for the elderly was started in Finsbury by the Employment Fellowship in conjunction with Finsbury Borough Council (as it was then). The Employment Fellowship is a voluntary organisation which gives help and advice in the setting up of work rooms in any part of the country where there is need for them. It will, in approved cases, give initial financial aid in the establishment of work rooms.

Since 1951, when the Fellowship began, eighty work rooms have been set up in such disparate places as Camden, Taunton and Huddersfield. The work rooms aim to provide elderly people with sheltered occupations which are not too physically demanding and at which they can work at their own steady pace. In most cases this is in the form of outwork from local industry and includes such tasks as folding trade circulars, sewing, sorting records and addressing envelopes. In some cases the work rooms make small household articles for direct sale.

Under the National Assistance Act 1948 (Amendment) Act, 1962, local authorities are empowered to maintain workshops for old people, either directly or through the agency of voluntary organisations. The majority of workshops are still run by voluntary committees, though often heavily subsidised by the local authority, and while there are financial advantages in direct control by the local authorities, it would be unfortunate if the voluntary element were eliminated or discouraged. Voluntary workers who devote their leisure time to the cause have always been of great advantage in the welfare of the centre and the workers. A voluntary committee can secure a charitable status in law and then obtain concessions relating to income tax, rates and entertainment duties on money raising events. Some schemes use the term 'workshop'.

EXPERIMENTS IN INDUSTRY AND COMMERCE

A few firms, notably Messrs Rubery Owen & Co Ltd, Engineers, The Crittall Manufacturing Company, and The John Lewis Partnership, Ltd, have pioneered new approaches to retirement for their employees. Work shops have been set up where employees may (if they wish) continue to work several hours a day at less arduous tasks; a few companies have reorganised their pension schemes on a flexible basis so that people could retire – voluntarily or otherwise – at any time after they reach fifty-five; other firms encourage their manual workers to taper off gradually during the later years of their employment and in some cases commercial concerns, such as banks and insurance offices, offer part-time work to their newly retired ex-employees at peak periods of the year. All these experiments have proved valuable and should stimulate other employers to reconsider their present policies on retirement and the use of the older worker. At present there are some fourteen known schemes run by firms for their retired employees.

PRE-RETIREMENT ADVISORY COURSES

Advisory courses, or discussion groups, have been run by over 260 organisations (mainly local education authorities), and are the principal concern of seventeen local preparation for retirement committees. Though people attending them are generally within a few months of finishing work, the courses are of most value to people with five or ten years still to go and who therefore have time to plan for the complete change in the pattern of living that retirement involves.

THE FINANCIAL IMPLICATIONS OF RETIREMENT

THE EARNINGS RULE

The earnings rule which was introduced by the National Insurance Act in 1946 is designed to reinforce the retirement principle. During the first five years after the minimum retirement age, pensioners in receipt of a state retirement pension are subject to the earnings rule, which means that deductions are made from the pension of those whose earnings per week exceed a prescribed sum. This sum now stands at £6 10s. a week, but allowances can be claimed for certain expenses, such as the cost of travelling to work, special clothing, and so on. The deductions made under the earnings rule are weighted against the worker as his earnings become larger: for the first £2 of earnings over £6 10s. sixpence is deducted from the pension for every shilling earned over £6 10s.; after that a shilling is deducted for every shilling earned over £8 10s. One result of this is that some pensioners decide to restrict their earnings below the prescribed sum per week and to seek part-time work so that their earnings supplement their income without affecting the amount of pension they receive.

SELECTIVE EMPLOYMENT TAX

The recently introduced Selective Employment Tax is not intended to discourage employers from taking on older or disabled workers. As there were some misgivings on this score further legislation was introduced in August, 1967. Now half the tax payable in respect of adult employees, normally working less than twenty-one hours a week in establishments not at present entitled to premium or refund, will in future be refunded. The measure is taken mainly because a number of part-time workers are elderly people who no longer want to work full-time but still have a useful contribution to make.

OCCUPATIONAL PENSION SCHEMES

An enquiry carried out by the Ministry of Pensions and National Insurance in 1966 discovered that nearly one half of the men surveyed (about 10,000) received some form of occupational pension on retirement. An increasing number of firms are arranging private pension schemes for their employees and therefore this proportion is bound to increase in the future. At present some occupational pension schemes discourage the employment of the older worker by specifying an age at which the pension must be drawn; there are also difficulties in admitting new employees over a certain age to the benefits of a scheme and in the transference of pension rights from one pension fund to another. While some occupational pension schemes tend to be inflexible in their approach to these matters, others have built-in modifications which minimise the difficulties of admitting newly employed older people and a few other positive incentives to defer retirement in the form of an ultimately higher pension.

Recent studies in the field have urged employers to adopt such modifications and incentives where possible so that their schemes can give the worker freedom of choice instead of imposing a rigid retirement pattern upon him.

REFERENCES

Circulars and other HMSO *Publications:*

Employment of Older Men and Women. Ministry of Labour National Advisory Committee report, 1953, HMSO, 2s 0d; Second report, 1955, HMSO, 1s 9d

The Older Worker and His Job. DSIR Booklet—Problems and Progress in Industry no 7, H. M. Clay, 1960, HMSO, 1s 3d

Ageing and the Semi-Skilled. A Survey in Manufacturing Industry on Merseyside. A. Heron and S. M. Chown, assisted by M. S. Featherstone and C. M. Cunningham. 1961, HMSO, 5s 0d

The Pattern of the Future. Ministry of Labour Manpower Study no 1. 1964, HMSO, 4s 0d

Everybody's Guide to Social Security. 1967, HMSO, 1s 0d

For further reading:

(*A*) NOPWC/NCSS *Publications:*

Employment and Workshops for the Elderly. 1963, 2s 0d

(*B*) *Other relevant publications:*

A Brief Guide to Pre-Retirement Advisory Courses. 1967, The Pre-Retirement Association, 2s 0d

Solving New Problems. A. Heron. 1963, Pre-Retirement Association, 2s 6d

Elderly Employed. D. Snellgrove. 1965, White Crescent Press, Luton, 10s 0d

Employment, Income and Retirement Problems of the Aged, edited by J. M. Kreps. 1964, Cambridge University Press, 60s 0d

Ageing and Human Skill, A. T. Welford. 1958, Nuffield Foundation, Oxford University Press, 25s 0d

Growing Old in a Mechanised World, F. le Gros Clark. 1960, Nuffield Foundation, 7s 6d

Work, Age and Leisure, F. le Gros Clark. 1966, Joseph, 30s 0d

Annual Reports and literature of the Employment Fellowship.

Not Too Old at Sixty. An experiment in the employment of women of pensionable age by the Over-Forty Association for Women. 1963, National Corporation for the Care of Old People, 2s 6d

Women, Work and Age, F. le Gros Clark. 1962, Nuffield Foundation, 7s 6d

Workrooms for the Elderly. PAS leaflet no 16. 1961, Rotary International, 6d

Age and Function, A Heron and S. Chown. 1967, J. & A. Churchill, 45s 0d

Job Re-Design and Occupational Training for Older Workers. Reports of the International Management Seminar. 1964, Organisation for Economic Co-operation and Development, Paris 1965, 15s 0d (*obtainable from* HMSO).

Workers Nearing Retirement. 1963, The Nuffield Foundation, 5s 0d

Useful Addresses:

The Employment Fellowship,
Drayton House, Gordon Street, London WC 1

Rotary International,
Sheen Lane House, Sheen Lane, London SW 14

Pre-Retirement Association,
35 Queen Anne Street, London W 1

Ministry of Labour,
8 St James's Square, London SW 1

CHAPTER EIGHT

The enjoyment and use of leisure

INTRODUCTORY

It is now a commonplace that the increasing amount of mechanisation and automation used in our industrial society will result in an increasing amount of leisure for our citizens. This change is beginning to affect all age groups, but its greatest effect is likely to be upon the elderly. One of the frequently adopted – though by no means entirely satisfactory – solutions to the over-employment problem is to dispense with the older worker. Though a worker often retires at a considerably earlier age than his forbears, his life expectancy is much longer than theirs ever was. He may, therefore, have a 'bonus' of ten to fifteen years of reasonably active life ahead of him. What should he do with it? This is a problem to be considered by both the individual and the community.

The processes of ageing must entail a certain amount of disengagement from what was a person's normal sphere of activity during the years of younger adulthood. The most decisive break with previous patterns occurs when elderly people retire from work and often tend to lose the sense of making a purposeful contribution to society which working life brings. There are other and related social factors which operate both before and after retirement, which make elderly people feel that they are expected to withdraw from full time involvement in the community. A woman whose time has been principally taken up with her family, finds that her children leave home and no longer need her constant care; people are often encouraged, and indeed wish, to reduce their working commitments and this may lead to less whole-hearted participation in business life. Some people, of course, stubbornly resist pressure to reduce their commitments or to believe that they are less capable at sixty-five of doing anything they could do at forty, but some diminution of physical and mental resources does occur and an ageing person finds eventually that he cannot function as speedily or efficiently as he once did, and that less work will be expected of him.

In addition, as people get older their circle of relatives and friends tends to diminish through death or long separation; in the case of those with families, a number of their social contacts come through their children and leave with them; working people miss the companionship of their colleagues; in these ways the sense of social isolation is frequently felt just at the time when people have more leisure and more desire and need to be sociable.

Ideally, then, leisure activities for the elderly perform two very valuable, very important functions: they help old people to regain or develop a sense of meaning and usefulness which they may have lost when the normal patterns of their everyday work are over; they give to those who need it, a renewed feeling of social participation and companionship – a filling of the gap left by a diminution of previous social relationships.

INDIVIDUAL PURSUITS – FOR PURPOSE AND PLEASURE

When considering leisure activities of elderly people, it is important to remember that great numbers of them have spent most of their life working either directly or indirectly for money. The simple business of getting in order to spend was in itself purpose enough, and it is difficult for them now to dissociate time spent from money earned. In retirement time needs to be given a purpose, which is seldom linked to direct financial reward.

WORK FOR THE COMMUNITY

Once a division between time and money has been accepted, numbers of elderly people find that they can put their abilities to very good use in the service of the community. Local voluntary organisations of all kinds need help – people to serve on their committees and organise events, to give practical help to those in need; to publicise their work and raise funds. Large numbers of old people's welfare committees are run by retired people who use their business and home-making skills to run the committee effectively and to give aid particularly to the frailer housebound old. Other voluntary organisations, particularly those which help the blind, deaf, the physically and the mentally handicapped depend a great deal on the service given by retired people. In such ways men and women can continue to use the particular talents they have acquired during their working lives: the ex-accountant who becomes a treasurer; the ex-electrician who mends appliances; the ex-teacher who gives talks of general interest; the ex-nurse who helps to care for the bedridden in a family emergency. In fact, any older person who is mobile and can do anything useful for someone else, cooking or driving, carpentry or writing, gardening or book-keeping, need never feel useless.

In addition to voluntary organisations, public bodies of various kinds use a great deal of voluntary service and those elderly who are interested in the affairs of the community at large should feel able to take an active interest in the general welfare of the people around them. The present movement to develop community care and good neighbourliness provides particular opportunity for the retired person.

LEARNING AND DEVELOPING

Words like learning and developing are invariably associated with the young, as if it were something only they did, but these processes go on throughout life and many elderly people use their leisure creatively by beginning new activities or perfecting that 'something they always wanted to do well, but never had time to'.

Learning something new

(1) *Courses for all age groups:* Local education authorities and organisations such as Townswomen's Guilds and the Workers' Educational Association, organise regular courses on a great variety of subjects – learning a new language for instance, training in cookery, carpentry, dress-making, appreciation courses in music or

literature. They are invariably open to people of all ages and cater for beginners as well as more advanced students. Details of courses in an area are available from public libraries, local education offices or citizens' advice bureaux.

(2) *Courses for older people:* A number of residential day courses especially for elderly people have been organised in recent years by old people's welfare committees and councils of social service in co-operation with local education authorities, the Workers' Education Association and extra-mural departments and colleges and universities. The courses aim to stimulate new interests such as local history, nature study, painting and also offer practical guidance to the elderly on, for example, how to protect one's health, cook on a small budget, guard against accidents. Residential courses are particularly valuable because they not only arouse new enthusiasms but provide opportunities for the elderly to make new friends and to introduce different kinds of elderly people to each other.

(3) *Preparation for Retirement Courses:* Pre-retirement advisory courses are provided by pre-retirement associations, commercial firms and local education bodies (*see* chapter Seven).

Developing interests

There are some enthusiasms such as for gardening, handicrafts, writing, knitting in which people have engaged for many years but have never pursued beyond a certain point. Many elderly people, who like to continue with what is already familiar, particularly enjoy a chance to improve a skill they already have. In addition to courses for more advanced students as mentioned above, old people's welfare committees, clubs and other voluntary organisations help to increase interest in these activities by organising competitions and exhibitions – competitions in essay writing or bulb growing for instance, exhibitions of art and handicraft. In some cases people find that they have attained sufficient skill to make their hobby a lucrative one: clay and pottery work, articles of embroidery, baskets, pictures – all these are saleable if the standard of work is reasonably good. Some elderly people use their hobbies to help the less able, by giving them to charity sales or by making useful articles for homes for old people or children, or refugee organisations.

Books of instruction on hobbies of all kinds can be obtained from public libraries and certain voluntary bodies, such as Women's Institutes, are always willing to give advice about handicrafts and domestic skills. For learning, entertainment and amusement books are always available and are a great source of comfort for many elderly. Libraries are very willing to help in selecting books if required and for the housebound many libraries make special arrangements to deliver books to the home. For those whose eyesight is failing, there is the series of Ulverscroft large print books, usually available from public libraries, and old people's welfare committees. Elderly people who find that they cannot read at all, can contact the local home teacher for the blind to advise on the possibility of learning braille or moon. Books for the blind can be obtained from the Royal National Institute for the Blind; there is also a library of talking books which can be borrowed (*for further details of these, see reference section at end of chapter*).

GROUP ACTIVITIES–FOR COMPANIONSHIP AND INTEREST

TYPES OF GROUPS

Special clubs for those over sixty are extremely popular with many of the older generation today. No record of the number of these clubs exists but it is thought that it cannot be less than 8,000. Clubs of all kinds have developed according to the needs and resources of the locality around them and the personalities of the people concerned with them. There are, therefore, a great number of variations on the theme of bringing together groups of old people and they differ enormously in intention, patterns of organisation and selection of priorities. The main sorts of clubs are as follows, but all old people's clubs and centres do not fall neatly into any one of these categories, all have an immense preventive value:

(1) *Day Clubs or Centres:* A club or centre of this kind, specifically for retired people, is extremely valuable to the elderly in the community. It sets out to provide warm, comfortable accommodation to which an old person can come during the day and meet friends and/or participate in various group activities. A mid-day meal is often provided, and indeed this is one of the most important facilities such a centre or club should offer. Sometimes a chiropody clinic also functions there and laundry equipment in some cases is available for members to do their personal washing. On the recreational side, handicrafts, choir, drawing and painting classes are very popular and local education authorities are generally only too willing to supply instructors if possible. Women's Institutes and Townswomen's Guilds can often help with teachers and equipment. Most day clubs and centres provide newspapers and library books and the bigger ones may have a TV room and a smoking/billiards room for the men.

There are many varieties of day clubs and centres. Some are run by an old people's welfare committee with help from its constituent bodies; others are the direct responsibility of one voluntary organisation such as the WRVS, BRCS, or local old age pensions association. There are now an increasing number provided by local authorities which, besides employing some paid staff, usually have the help of voluntary workers. All daily clubs and centres have their own premises, though some are only rented. Many are purpose-built. There is also a wide variety in the way the day club or centre is run. Some are open to any local retired person without membership fee; others limit the use of the premises to those who have joined the club or centre. The term 'club' is used in some cases; 'centre', 'drop-in-centre', 'all-day centre', or just a name such as 'Alfriston' describes others. There is no set rule in the organisation or scope of these daily clubs or centres; each follows its own pattern, developed according to the resources available and the needs of the local elderly people. Many elderly people play an invaluable part in helping to run a daily club or centre.

(2) *Non-daily clubs:* As the name implies, these clubs meet regularly, once or twice weekly, fortnightly, or even monthly. The non-daily clubs normally meet in hired premises, that is, church or

village halls or rooms belonging to the Scouts, British Legion or local authority, etc. There is nearly always a membership system with subscriptions (often very small) for these clubs and very many of them are independent of any organisation and are run by the members themselves. Others are run by old people's welfare committees, voluntary organisations and churches, and club members help in the management. Some clubs have a very wide range of activities and facilities; others have limited programmes. The latter naturally appeal to a smaller proportion of the elderly community than the first.

Clubs having subscribing members vary enormously in their total membership; they can be as small as twenty or go to 250 or more. The large structured clubs tend to be more organised and to cater for particular social groups; the smaller ones to be more informal both regarding activities and membership.

(3) *Lunch and Dinner Clubs:* Many day and some non-daily clubs provide their members with a good, hot, cheap mid-day meal. There are, however, some clubs which are held only for the purpose of offering lunch on one or more days a week to the members. The work of preparing the meals may be undertaken by a rota of women's organisations or by one group of volunteers, often greatly helped by the members of the club. The meals are usually cooked on the premises and sometimes the cook may be paid. Members are charged the full cost of the meal where expenses are not high; sometimes the cost of the meal is subsidised by the local authority or from voluntary sources so as to keep the charge low. Old people greatly appreciate not having to prepare their own meal for one or two days a week and also enjoy the change of eating with others. Care should be taken in planning nutritious as well as appetising meals in a lunch club because adequate diet plays an important part in preventing deterioration, both in physical and mental health.

Quite often a luncheon club will gradually enlarge its scope to include various group activities for the afternoon and will develop into an ordinary social club for the elderly.

(4) *Day Centres and Clubs for housebound and handicapped old*

people: Some areas concentrate on the specific needs of physically and/or mentally handicapped old people and provide day centres specially for them, others where numbers are small, include them in ordinary day centres. This is a particularly important and valuable task, for such people tend to be the most isolated in the community and greatly appreciate companionship and a change of surroundings. In addition to providing meals and certain group activities, in which members are able to participate, the day centre arranges transport to and from the club and extra facilities such as bathing, hairdressing and chiropody. Members usually come regularly and stay the whole day at the club once a week. This helps also to relieve the burden on those who look after the old person for the rest of the time, or to alleviate the monotony of those who live alone.

For those old people who suffer from blindness, deafness or a crippling physical handicap there are special clubs catering for these infirmities in many places.

(5) *Special Interest Clubs:* There is no reason, of course, why the elderly should be expected to only join clubs for members of their own age groups. Most towns of any size contain groups which meet to pursue their own particular enthusiasms – for photography, local history, bee-keeping, drama, etc. Many elderly enjoy maintaining and expanding interests in these special fields and developing through them their links with the rest of the community. Sometimes, too, a few elderly people within a large group will form a special interest group and arrange activities such as choir concerts or art exhibitions. Community centres cater admirably for retired people as they provide interesting classes and hobby groups for all ages, and many of them also run a special social group for men and women over sixty.

CLUBS FOR THE ELDERLY – ORGANISATION

Full information about the setting-up and administration of clubs is given in the National Old People's Welfare Council's handbook *Leisure in Later Years* (*see further reference section at the end of this chapter*).

(a) *Constitution*

Independent clubs (that is those not administered by a body such as the Women's Royal Voluntary Service or the British Red Cross Society) will need to adopt a constitution. The National Old People's Welfare Council has drawn up a model which has been accepted by the Charity Commission and the Inland Revenue. Those clubs owning their premises and/or with an annual income above a certain level should register as a charity with the Charity Commission. (See *Leisure in Later Years,* p. 75.)

(b) *Finance*

(1) *Statutory grants:* Local authorities have power under the *National Assistance Act, 1948 (Amendment) Act 1962* to give financial assistance to a voluntary body providing a club for the elderly by an initial grant towards capital expenditure and/or an annual grant towards the upkeep of the club. They can also make available land for building or premises to house the club without charge or at a low rental. The majority of local authorities exercise these powers to a varying degree. In return the club itself is expected to raise part of the money needed and it must be able to give a satisfactory account of the way in which the local authority grant is used.

Section 4 of the Physical Training and Recreation Act, 1937, permits all local authorities (including parish councils) to make grants to schemes with a substantial 'social and educational' content. This power is used chiefly where an old people's club is part of a community centre or association.

(2) *Grants from voluntary sources:* The National Old People's Welfare Council administers a small fund, placed at its disposal by Unilever Ltd, to help clubs and centres with small purchases of equipment or furniture. Forms of application are available from secretaries of county or county borough old people's welfare committees.

Local voluntary organisations, such as Rotary, Toc H and Round Table are often generous in helping clubs. Also local charitable trusts may sometimes exist which could help an old people's club. Such trusts are listed with the local authority. A club's income is also built up by membership fees, profit on sales of refreshments, hand work and bring-and-buy sales, entertainments, raffles, etc.

(c) *Insurance*
Clubs are well advised to have good insurance cover. A special insurance scheme with a favoured rate for premiums for public liability and personal accident insurance cover is available for those clubs not covered by any parent organisation. Premises and property should also be covered against fire, damage, etc. Full details and advice are available from the National Old People's Welfare Council.

(d) *Rates*
Under the Rating and Valuation Act, 1961, an institution qualifying as of charitable status and using its premises wholly or mainly for charitable purposes will be entitled as of right to fifty per cent relief from rates, and in addition a rating authority will have power, if they wish, to reduce or remit the balance. (*See Leisure in Later Years,* p. 76).

(e) *Forget-me-not badges*
Many clubs for the elderly use these badges as their emblem. This gives them a feeling of belonging to a larger movement and when they join in holiday schemes or rallies they are able to recognise other club members if they wear the forget-me-not badge. These can be obtained from the National Old People's Welfare Council.

CLUB ACTIVITIES
The range of club activities depends on the capability and the inclinations of its members, the amount of initiative shown by its organisers, its financial resources and the resources of the locality. Some of the principally popular activities are as follows:

Music: Most old people enjoy singing, dancing, playing music and listening to it. Club choirs are very popular and they often entertain other groups in the district and enter competitions.

Handicrafts and Hobbies: Some people prefer to pursue their handicraft hobbies outside a club (*see above*) but many benefit from the stimulation of group activity. Classes or informal groupings for dressmaking, rugmaking, woodwork, model photography and embroidery are all popular in clubs. Classes in painting and drawing are growing in popularity and aspiring writers often benefit from group discussion of their work and especially enjoy writing their youthful memories. Drama is, of course, essentially a group activity and once members are helped to feel that they are capable of taking part, amateur dramatics usually go well. For all these activities a club is well advised to contact outside sources of help – art and drama teachers from schools, other local societies, librarians for instance. Members interested in these activities can also be stimulated by the organising of exhibitions and competitions at both national and local levels.

Entertainment of general interest: Films can be hired or borrowed from a number of sources (*see further reference section*) and technical advice on showing them can be obtained from local photographic societies or education authorities. Film strips are easier to show and cheaper but frequently need amplification by a speaker. The range of subjects for talks to clubs is limitless. Some which are particularly popular with elderly people are: gardening, health and diet, travel, local history, religious talks, surveys of statutory services. Speakers can be found among local professional people, members of other groups and members of the club itself. Some old people who do not have television may enjoy the chance to see it at the club. Tape recorders are being increasingly used by club leaders to record the dialects of local people, for example, or talks, concerts and plays given at the club itself.

Games, Collecting, Competitions: Games such as billiards, draughts, darts and collecting things, such as coins and stamps, are particularly popular with men and if facilities for these activities can be provided, male membership usually increases. Whist, scrabble, bridge and dominoes are popular with everyone. Competitions in connection with these activities arouse friendly rivalry as do other competitions such as for growing bulbs, baking cakes, arranging flowers.

Christmas parties, day outings to the seaside or places of special interest: These are always popular. Some clubs organise group holidays for their members and this is very valuable, particularly if help is concentrated on the frailer members (even perhaps the semi-housebound) who cannot themselves cope with travel arrangements.

Spreading Information: A most important function of a club is to pass on useful information to its members. This can be done in several ways: by inviting experts such as dietitians, Ministry of Social Security officers, health visitors to speak on their particular speciality; by displaying leaflets and notices about pensions, rate rebates, local authority services and so on on the club notice board and by producing a regular club bulletin in which such details can be published. Items of national interest are mentioned in the *Quarterly Bulletin* of the National Old People's Welfare Council and can always be reproduced by clubs.

REFERENCES

Circulars and HMSO Publications:

Physical Training and Recreation Act, 1937. HMSO, 1s 6d
Local Government Act, 1948. HMSO, 7s 6d
Rating and Valuation Act, 1961. HMSO, 3s 0d
National Assistance Act, 1948. (Amendment) Act, 1962. HMSO, 6d

For further reading:

(*A*) NOPWC/NCSS *Publications:*

Leisure in Later Years. 1963, 2s 6d
Clubs for the Elderly. 1966, 3s 6d
Model Constitution for Clubs. Free
Handicrafts for Older People. 1963, 6d
The Over Sixties Club and the Community. 1964, *Free*
List of Talking Points for Small Discussion Groups. 1966, *Free*
Visual Aid Material concerned with the Care of the Elderly. A list. 1967, 6d

(*B*) *Other Relevant Publications:*

Leisure Activities for the Elderly. Obtainable from 'Home This Afternoon', BBC; 1967, *Free*
Enjoying Retirement, P. Shaw. 1961, Industrial Welfare Society, 2s 6d
Retire and Enjoy It, C. Chisholm. 1954, Penguin Books, 3s 6d

Lunch Clubs for the Elderly. Lancashire OPWC, Selnec House, Wynnstay Grove, Manchester 14, 1966, 2s 6d

Education and Retirement, B. Groombridge. 1960, National Institute of Adult Education, 8s 6d

Work, Age and Leisure, F. le Gros Clark. 1966, Michael Joseph, 50s 0d

Home This Afternoon, edited by J. Singleton. 1966, Lutterworth Press, 21s 0d

Something to be Done at Home, E. Gilzean. 1963, Museum Press. 12s 6d

Penguin Spare Time Book, T. Gibson and J. Singleton. 1961, Penguin, 3s 6d

Committee Procedure for Clubs and Voluntary Organisations, P. du Sautoy. 1963, Practical Books Series, Oxford University Press, 2s 0d

The Years Still Unexplored, F. le Gros Clark and F. S. Milligan. 1964, Pre-Retirement Association, 3s 6d

Creative Living. The Work and Purposes of a Community Association. National Federation of Community Associations, NCSS, 1964, 6s 0d

Voluntary Organisations and the Law Relating to Lotteries and Gaming. 1967, NCSS 3s 0d

Educating Older People, M. F. Cleugh. 1963, Tavistock Publications, 28s 0d

Useful Addresses:

Ulverscroft Large Print Books,
Station Road, Glenfield, Leicester

Workers' Educational Association,
27 Portman Square, London W 1

Royal National Institute for the Blind,
224 Great Portland Street, London W 1

National Library for the Blind,
35 Great Smith Street, London SW 1

Library Association,
Ridgemount Street, London WC 1

WRVS (Headquarters),
17 Old Park Lane, London W 1

National Institute of Adult Education,
35 Queen Anne Street, London W 1

National Federation of Community Associations,
26 Bedford Square, London WC 1

National Association of Women's Clubs,
26 Bedford Square, London WC 1

Charity Commission (registration division),
14 Ryder Street, London SW 1

CHAPTER NINE

Research and information

The justification for any social research is that the results help towards a better understanding of what is going on in society, and thus enable human problems to be met more satisfactorily. Whether such work is done on a national or a local basis, its value lies in that it presents parts of a changing picture from which the whole may be pieced together. In view of continual change in the many factors affecting the lives of the elderly – the value of money, population trends and distribution, slum clearance, new housing, changing attitudes to the ageing process and to the elderly themselves and many others – the importance of making available up-to-date information becomes obvious. By keeping and constantly revising this type of information, some purposeful attempt can be made to keep social policy in line with the needs brought to light in this way, and necessary pointers given for the shaping of policies for the future.

To be of value research must be carefully planned. Its objectives must be clearly defined and it must be carried out under the guidance of those who have mastered the necessary skills and techniques. Before embarking upon any kind of survey researchers should be quite sure that it will make a measurable contribution to the total body of information already available both in this country and overseas on the subject of human ageing, its social implications and the needs of the elderly. They must also make certain that there are sufficient funds available to cover the cost of the research and sufficient time for the workers concerned to complete their job properly. Results obtained must be reliable and should be explained in such a way as to be intelligible to those who are likely to seek knowledge and guidance from them. It should also be noted that survey results even when obtained by qualified research workers using accredited techniques are still sometimes open to misinterpretation. If survey results have sufficient value for either a lay reader or a professional group to warrant publication then they should be published as soon as possible. Out of date material is of little use.

In general, research into human ageing and its social effects is making a greater use of scientific investigatory techniques. There is also a growing awareness of how the study of the ageing process and its social implications interacts with many other disciplines – such as biology, sociology, psychology.

The growing realisation that research into the social field of ageing is necessary and valuable has resulted in the undertaking of a considerably increased number of projects in recent years. These studies vary a great deal in their scope, purpose and overall quality. In order to keep in touch with them the National Old People's Welfare Council set up an Advisory Group on Surveys and Research. In 1960 the group prepared *A Short Guide to Social Survey Methods.*

The proliferation of material revealed the need for a register of the research carried out in the social and socio-medical fields of old people's welfare in order to disseminate knowledge already accumulated and to prevent overlapping. In 1960, therefore, the National Corporation for the Care of Old People published its first *Old Age – a Register of Social Research.* In 1964 the National Corporation for the Care of Old People published a bound edition for the years 1955-1964; this has been followed by further annual supplements. Those who intend to initiate or take part in research in the social field of ageing are advised to consult the register and to contact the National Old People's Welfare Council's Advisory Group for information and advice.

THE NATURE OF SOCIAL SURVEYS

A social survey aims to collect facts about the social aspects of a community – that is the way in which people affect and are affected by the wider society in which they live. Facts are usually obtained by putting carefully framed impartial questions directly to the members of the group which is being studied. The assembled answers to these questions can invariably be expressed in quantitative terms. The aims of social surveys are mostly utilitarian. With regard to research into the welfare of the elderly this means that investigators try to learn more about practical social problems which affect their position in the community.

Surveys differ tremendously in their scope and aims according to who is carrying them out. For example, those conducted by Ministries tend to be framed in such a way so that indications of national trends and predictions of general social patterns can be made from them. Other surveys are conducted on a purely local scale and results from them are intended to be relevant only to the particular local circumstances.

Observations collected may be purely descriptive in content (for example how many old people in a certain city live with their children); they may seek to find an explanation for a particular situation (for example the reasons for entry into residential homes of elderly people in a certain area); they may seek to assess possible future implications of a particular social phenomenon (for example the post-retirement physical fitness and psychological attitudes of a group of men who continue to work up to the age of 70). Sometimes the whole of a limited specified group is surveyed (for example all patients over 60 admitted to a particular mental hospital during a certain period). In other cases a sample is selected for study and is picked so as to be as representative as possible of a larger group.

RESEARCH TECHNIQUES

LONGITUDINAL METHODS

In this method investigators usually take a sample of the relevant population and obtain information from them by means of personal interviews. At regular intervals of perhaps a year or two years these same people are again interviewed – either directly or by post. The results obtained are calculated on each occasion and researchers are then able to measure precisely how a particular section of the population has developed over the years and reacted to varying circumstances. One outstanding advantage of this technique is that the respondents are not asked to try and remember their earlier circumstances – these are already known to the researcher.

POINT OF TIME METHOD

In such studies investigators select samples of subjects who are comparable in many respects and by interviews ascertain their circumstances and attitudes at the time when the survey is being carried out. There is always the risk here that the information collected will soon become out of date – another risk is that the information may be affected by the time of the year when the research is carried out – for example, needs and attitudes may well be different in summer than in winter.

THE NATIONAL OLD PEOPLE'S WELFARE COUNCIL AND RESEARCH

The National Old People's Welfare Council's Advisory Group on surveys and research meets twice yearly. Its purpose is to assess material already published in order to inform and advise the Council, and to decide upon its wider dissemination; to keep the Council informed of work in progress and future projects contemplated, and to offer advice to those undertaking surveys if this is sought. The Council itself, in consultation with the group and other organisations, encourages research in those areas of old people's welfare where more informed study is required.

Every three years the National Old People's Welfare Council carries out by post a survey which assesses the extent of the services provided for the elderly in the United Kingdom by voluntary organisations. Old people's welfare committees throughout the country are circulated with a questionnaire to be completed by committee secretaries. A report of the survey is produced for circulation to committees and other interested bodies and as a source of reference for researchers. In general terms the Council maintains continuous liaison with such bodies as the National Corporation for the Care of Old People, the European Research Section of the International Association of Gerontology and with various University Departments to keep abreast of, and participate in, new research developments.

REFERENCES

NOPWC/NCSS Publications:

A Short Guide to Social Survey Methods. 1960, 2s 6d

Reports of the NOPWC. Three-Yearly Survey of Voluntary Services for the Elderly.

Other Relevant Publications:

Old Age—A Register of Social Research. National Corporation for the Care of Old People, 1955-1964, 12s 6d; and 1964 onwards, £1 including future supplements

Survey Methods in Social Investigations, C. A. Moser. 1958, Heinemann, 35s 0d

The Tools of Social Science, J. Madge. 1963, Longmans, 15s 0d

Interviewing in the Social Services, E. & K. de Schweinitz. 1962, The National Institute for Social Work Training, NCSS, 4s 6d

Research in the Personal Social Services. National Institute for Social Work Training. 1965, NCSS, 2s 6d

Useful Addresses:

The National Corporation for the Care of Old People,
Nuffield Lodge, Regent's Park, London NW 1

Social Science Research Council,
State House, High Holborn, London WC 1

Appendix

HEALTH SERVICES AND PUBLIC HEALTH BILL, 1967

Clauses which may affect the elderly (or organisations working on their behalf) are given below as summarised in the Explanatory and Financial Memorandum prefacing the Bill.

'*The purpose of the Bill is to amend and supplement existing legislation in order to promote miscellaneous improvements in the health and welfare services, and the public health services.*

'Clause 11 *extends the power of local health authorities similarly to allow health visitors and nurses to attend patients elsewhere than in their homes.*

'Clause 13 *replaces existing provisions relating to the domestic help service. It makes it a duty for local health authorities to provide this service, and empowers them to make available laundry facilities as a part of it.*

'Clauses 29 and 30 *enable the Minister to allow services (e.g. laundry facilities) and goods (e.g. surgical dressings, artificial eyes) in excess of the requirements of the hospital service to be used outside the service, on such terms as he may determine, and to provide such services and goods in excess of the requirements of the Hospital Service.*

'Clause 42 *enables local authorities to accommodate the elderly and the handicapped in registered homes run privately for profit, as well as in local authority or voluntary homes as at present.*

'Clause 43 *enables authorities to make arrangements, subject to the Minister's approval, to promote the welfare of the elderly, and empowers the Minister to direct them to do so. This will enable authorities to develop "preventive welfare" for the elderly generally, in a similar manner to their power and duties in respect of the handicapped of all ages.*

'Clause 60 *puts on a statutory basis the present practice whereby the Minister gives financial assistance to voluntary organisations in the health and welfare field.*

'Clause 61 *consolidates and extends the powers of local authorities to give financial and other assistance to similar voluntary organisations.*'

Index

Publications are not included in this Index as they are listed at the end of each relevant chapter.